CALL AN AMBULANCE!

First edition, published in 2000 by

WOODFIELD PUBLISHING
Woodfield House, Babsham Lane, Bognor Regis
West Sussex PO21 5EL, England.

© Alan Crosskill, 2000

All rights reserved.
No part of this publication may be reproduced
or transmitted in any form or by any means,
electronic or mechanical, nor may it be stored
in any information storage and retrieval system,
without prior permission from the publisher.

ISBN 1-873203-63-2

CALL AN AMBULANCE!

Humorous recollections of a former Ambulanceman

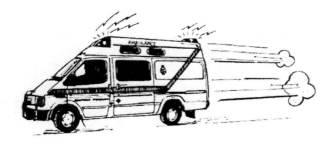

ALAN CROSSKILL

Woodfield Publishing
BOGNOR REGIS • WEST SUSSEX • ENGLAND

Acknowledgements

This book is dedicated to the committed, and often neglected, men and women of the NHS Ambulance Service - past and present.

May I record my special appreciation for help, inspiration and support to:

Guy Crosskill

Alan Duffy

Brian Fox

and my patient and long suffering wife

Illustrations kindly provided by Ged Wild at Richmond Ambulance Station Tees, East & North Yorkshire Ambulance Service NHS Trust

The incidents portrayed in this book are based on real events but the characters portrayed are entirely fictitious. Any resemblance to persons either living or dead is entirely coincidental.

Alan Crosskill
April 2000

Contents

Preface 7
PROLOGUE: The Driving Test 9
1. Joining Up 15
2. The First Day 26
3. Uniform Issue 36
4. Plug in the Standby Crew 45
5. Sex and escorts 53
6. Blooded 60
7. Mental Patients 68
8. Jack's Tea 74
9. The Greatcoat 82
10. It could happen to anyone 88
11. The Docks 96
12. Change 102
13. More Changes 109
14. The Explosion 117

15.	Working together	123
16.	The Steel Works	131
17.	Risk to life and limb	140
18.	The Faux-Pas	147
19.	The Ambulance Drove Away	154
20.	Promotion	160
21.	Pheasants	167
22.	The Maternity	177
23.	The Wrong One	186
24.	Pheasants II	195
25.	The Bill	200
26.	Brazil Nuts	208
27.	China Tea	214
28.	Bathrooms	219
29.	Helping the Police	227
30.	Horses for Courses	234
31.	The Dog	240

Preface

Like the majority of my generation, I was a reluctant National Serviceman: I moaned from the day of call-up until demob, wanting to go back to civvie street where I belonged, and when I got back I was unsettled, wanting to do something interesting. Eventually I joined the ambulance service and 27 years later they let me retire with a pension and lots of memories.

Ambulance crews experience every misery befalling human beings; you name it, they deal with it. Someone once said to me, "How do you cope? I expect you get hardened." No, you don't get hardened! If you did, you would fail as ambulance crew. Ambulance staff need compassion and respect for people to do their job.

In my day they had not invented 'stress' – you just got on with the job or resigned! We managed by forgetting bad experiences, pushing them from our minds. At other times we saw the funny side, and it's these experiences, perhaps not funny at the time (often not for the patients) which I relate in this book. It is my attempt to give an intimation of life as an 'ambulanceman' before they invented 'paramedics', and it is to those highly skilled Paramedics and Technicians of the modern NHS Ambulance Service – men and women I so greatly admire – that this book is respectfully dedicated.

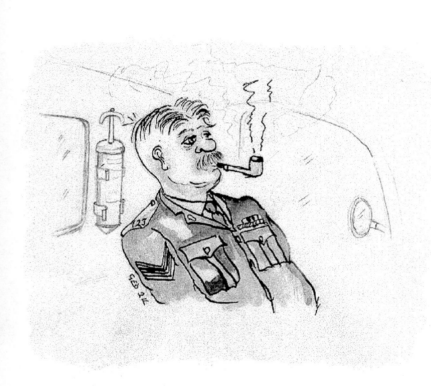

PROLOGUE

The Driving Test

My heart pounded, I went cold, my breathing stopped. Fleetingly, I closed my eyes and prayed, anticipating the crunch of metal on metal at any moment. Opening my eyes, I hastily glanced into the wing mirror and was surprised to see that I'd missed the lamppost with an inch to spare. I gulped, feeling my shirt sticking to my back and glanced across at my passenger. If he'd noticed anything at all, he gave no indication of it and continued his dreary dissertation, puffing non-stop at his foul-smelling pipe. My panic turned to anger. Did I have to put up with these pipe fumes? Did I *really* need this job so much? Yes I did!

Sod him. Somehow I would master the vehicle!

Reflecting back to that cold February day in 1965 makes me realise how much I've changed over the years. There's nothing like being an ambulanceman to knock off the rough edges of callow youth. On that morning I was a very youthful, very apprehensive and rather naive ex-soldier taking my driving test for a job as an ambulanceman. I'd had the interview and medical and had been rather surprised and filled with awe that the police would conduct the driving test. Needless to say I was more than a little nervous when reporting to the ambulance station at the appointed hour, I was shown to the seemingly huge white Bedford ambulance.

Sitting alone in the cab, staring at the enormous white snooker table of a bonnet, I recall feeling on edge, a bundle of nerves, convinced I would never cope, never control anything so large without hitting something! Everything about the vehicle looked huge. I'd been so keen to get the job that the size of the vehicle I would be required to handle in traffic had never occurred to me.

My worries and thoughts as I sat high behind the steering wheel were interrupted as a rotund police sergeant with a bright red face, sweeping walrus moustache and bulbous nose, came into my field of vision. The policeman, on a large black bicycle, a folded police cape strapped to the handlebars, peddled sedately into the yard. Braking, he swung his leg over the saddle and with a hop and skip dismounted. With great care, he propped his steed against the wall, carefully removing the front light and placing it into the saddlebag. Turning towards the ambulance, the policeman stood, studying me for what seemed an age, the back of his hand repeatedly sweeping across that magnificent ginger moustache. Very carefully and slowly he removed his cycle clips, slipped them into his trouser pocket and walked deliberately towards the vehicle. After taking only a few paces he stopped, removed his helmet and wiped his brow with a large red spotted handkerchief. In stark contrast to that moustache, the sergeant's hair was jet black, cropped high and parted in the centre. Ponderously, he walked to the near side of the vehicle, opening the cab door and with much grunting and puffing, struggled up the high step into the cab where he collapsed back on to the seat, wheezing noisily to regain his breath after his exertions. Gradually the noise of his breathing became a little more controlled, but still alarming to my then untrained ears. After what seemed an age, and still without a word, the sergeant placed his helmet on the cab floor and started to pat the bulging pockets of his tunic, eventually pulling out a large and well-worn pipe, together with an old brass lighter. Wiping the stem of the pipe against his tunic cuff, he put the pipe into his mouth and sucked firmly, like a small child with a stick of rock. With great care he flicked the wheel of the lighter with a gnarled thumb until the thing erupted into a massive oily flame. He then proceeded to light the pipe. His cheeks worked in and out as he puffed hard, repeatedly pressing his finger onto the burning tobacco until the pipe was lit to his satisfaction. This was obviously an art-form to him, a ritual developed over many years. At last, as the cab filled with foul smoke, the sergeant settled back into the seat, contentedly puffing away. After about a minute he took the smelly object out of his mouth and, with the back of his other hand, swept his moustache back into its carefully groomed shape. He looked across at me and beamed.

"Ow do lad, Sar'nt Parker. When you're ready lad, off we go."

I had watched him perform his ritual in amazement, rather like a rabbit mesmerised by a stoat, but the sergeant's deep voice brought me back to reality. His period of silence had ended. Leaning forward the policeman studied me closely; I began to feel twinges of alarm. The deep voice boomed again.

"You ex-army son?"

I nodded and said 'Third Hussars, tank crew'.

An expression of pleasure spread across the sergeant's shiny red face. Proudly he tapped the double row of ribbons on his tunic with the stem of his pipe.

"I were a Tanky in the last lot. By gum it were nobut rough. I remember the time..."

With that he settled himself back into the seat and launched into a rambling anecdote about the desert campaign in North Africa. As I listened to him, I could almost feel the sand between my toes and hear the shells exploding around me. As he spoke he continued to puff at that foul smelling pipe, filling the cab with its acrid smoke.

I sat in silence listening to the monologue, but after some minutes I felt I ought to do something, so starting the engine we lurched and juddered out of the yard. In a similar fashion I drove around town, the vehicle making loud noises of protest as each gear change was crunched. I was disappointed and annoyed that all my efforts seemed of no great interest to the sanguine sergeant. Puffing contentedly at his pipe, pausing only to re-light it, he talked and reminisced; he had obviously enjoyed his war. The smoke in the cab soon became quite oppressive, but he had chosen to ignore my coughs and when I wound the window down an inch he hunched his shoulders and grumbled about a draught. I wanted the job, so I shut the window and suffered.

For the whole of the journey, the sergeant continued his musings, obviously pleased to have a captive audience. As he had given no instructions regarding where to go, I cautiously drove around a quiet ring road and back to the Ambulance Station. Pointing the massive bonnet and wings of the Bedford at the narrow gate and hoping I'd get in without too much damage to vehicle and wall the ambulance lurched back into its home.

Sweating, and not daring to attempt to reverse into the garage in which it had stood when I had arrived, I parked, more or less near the kerb, and switched off the engine. The sudden silence brought the sergeant back to reality. He sat up and looked around in amazement, eyes blinking, nose glowing.

"Are we back so soon? That were a lovely smooth ride, I did enjoy it! It were right grand. Been a pleasure to be with you lad and talk to thee. I'll go and tell 'em you've passed."

The policemen made no effort to move, settling back in his seat a faraway look returned to his eyes. His nicotine stained fingers caressed the shiny smooth surface of his lighter. Crossing one leg over the other, exposing a length of white long-john above a highly polished boot, the Sargent closed his eyes.

"The best bit though were when we went into Alexandria..."

He was oblivious to everything again, lost amid the desert sands, the shriek and rattle of tank tracks, reliving his youth. I silently opened the cab door and slid out. The man had said I'd passed the driving test so it seemed a shame to disturb his reminiscences.

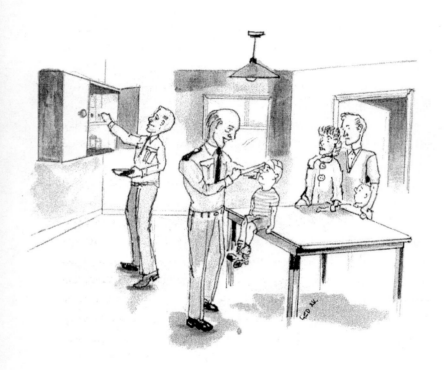

CHAPTER ONE

Joining Up

The plaintive crying of the solitary small boy lying on the ground made us hurry over to him. The youngster, about eight years old, had a nasty gash on the top of his head, and like all scalp wounds it was bleeding profusely. It was clear that he'd fallen from one of those metal climbing frames that local councils, in those days, thoughtfully bedded into solid concrete in the children's play areas of public parks.

I was in the park with my wife and small son, enjoying the late summer sunshine whilst the lad played on the swings and other amusements. Suddenly, like many people faced with an accident situation, I realised that I had no idea of what to do. Between his sobs the distressed child told us what had happened and where he lived, so consoling him, my wife and I put him in the car and took him home. In addition to our concern for him I wondered how I would remove the bloodstains from the plastic upholstery of my small and old car.

With some searching we at last found the house in a small shabby street off the market place, we were both horrified to find all was in darkness and locked, with no answer to our frantic knocking. A feeling of panic started to grow within me, I was well aware I was out of my depth. Suddenly, I remembered seeing an ambulance station down a side street not far away, so bundling the family and the snivelling boy back into the car we made our way to the ambulance station and escorted him into the office.

Like most people, I knew absolutely nothing about the Ambulance Service, apart from being aware that ambulances were large white things that I had seen going up and down the road. As soon as we entered the office with the boy, two uniformed men cheerfully took over. We were both relieved and impressed. The Ambulancemen chatted to the lad and soon calmed him as they bandaged his head. By the time they took him out to the ambulance and on to the hospital, he was chattering to them like old friends. As they went out, one of the drivers winked at me and said that the lad would be all right. I well believed him. The whole incident made me think, and, as it turned out, that boy's accident completely changed my life.

Like most young men of that era, on attaining the age of eighteen I had served two years as a National Serviceman, reluctantly obeying the government's demand that all young males undertake two years military service. Like many millions of others I had found myself in a strange new world composed of khaki, blanco, NCOs with loud voices, hard boots, hours of marching up and down a seemingly endless barrack square and nights spent 'guarding' large expanses of the wild and empty moorland areas of North Yorkshire. After basic and trade training I was posted to an armoured regiment in Germany, where I reluctantly admit that I enjoyed the majority of my service as part of a tank crew.

On demobilisation I was not alone in finding that the freedom of civvie street and returning to a boring job soon palled after my spell of Army life. Not, mark you, enough to make me think of reenlisting, but just enough to make me think about a change of career. The realisation of how little I knew about helping others in need, a desire to do something worthwhile, coupled with a yearning to become part of a uniformed organisation again, attracted me to the Ambulance Service.

A few months later my wife pointed out an advert in the local paper:

> Men required to drive the County Council's ambulances and render first aid if required. £12.6.4 per week. Uniform provided. Apply to...

The pay was awful, but the more I though about it, the more I wanted to join. I wanted to belong to an organisation again, and more importantly I wanted a worthwhile job. Once the idea had formed in my mind and I knew I had my wife's support, I couldn't wait to join. Taking the initiative, I made an appointment to visit the Ambulance Station and talk to the Station Officer.

Mr Green was delighted to see a potential recruit, especially one who appeared so keen. He eyed me up and down whilst I stood erectly before his desk. Although I had no way of knowing, the fact that I was in my very early twenties, smart, slim and fit and had served in the Army, went well in my favour in Mr Green's eyes.

Station Officer James Green, a short dumpy man, was a great believer in the old saying 'youth is wasted on the young.' I later learnt that he was constantly reminded by his wife that he was overweight. Below his bald pate and fringe of sandy coloured hair shone a bright red face, always looking as though it had just been scrubbed – "Like a turkey cock's arse" – I later heard a member of staff describe it. Pebble lens glasses magnified his beady eyes, and as always his station officer's navy blue uniform was well pressed, looking very smart with silver buttons and two stars on each shoulder. Unblinking, I returned his stare. I had already guessed that this was a man full of his own importance – a 'bullshitter'.

Green leaned back in his chair, smiled benevolently at me and proceeded to live up to my initial estimate by giving a lot of bull and flannel about the Service. The man made the job sound far better than it was and made himself appear to be very important, leading me to believe that he had saved more lives than I'd had hot dinners. In addition, he left me with the impression that I would be rushing attractive young damsels in see-through nylon nightdresses into hospital on a daily basis and with an exaggerated wink, he intimated that pretty nurses would be falling over themselves to get to know a smart young chap like me! Of course, by then, I had forgotten my first impression and was willing to believe him. As an ex-squaddie, I believed everyone with pips on their shoulder. At that age many young men tend to be naive.

In due course I was overjoyed to be called for interview at County Hall, they even sent me a free rail ticket, although the fact appeared to have been overlooked that, following a wide-reaching review of the railways by a certain Doctor Beeching, the town no longer had a railway station!

At the required time and date, polished, and pressed, I presented myself for interview. I'd never been to County Hall before and was most impressed by the huge Victorian building in the heart of the county town. Reporting to a uniformed commissioner at the reception desk, I was directed to the Health Department. After the first half mile of corridors and turnings I was totally lost. Becoming desperate, I asked a rather plain young girl for directions. She enquired why I wanted to go there. When I told her it was for a job interview, she insisted on taking me. As I followed her skinny figure I soon became certain that I could never have found the department on my own. The teenage girl, who was remarkably unattractive, chattered non-stop as we walked. I learned a little about the County Council and an awful lot about her, where she worked, her hobbies and interests. I took little notice of her or what she had to say apart from thinking to myself how boring it would be to work with her for long. In my excitement I was too ignorant to realise that I was being 'chatted up'!

The girl at last left me at the Health Department with a reminder of her name and the department she worked in; facts which I immediately forgot. Tapping on the door, I entered the office. The large room was full of desks, each occupied by a male or female clerk, every desk and available workspace cluttered with piles of papers, large books and bulging folders. No one took any notice of me; everyone concentrated on writing frantically. They must have been very busy.

Just as I was about to ask for directions, a very large and rather frightening lady, looking very much like my old sergeant major, marched into the room, bore down on me. She had the presence of one who was used to being obeyed. I was immediately terrified, being still of an age to be frightened by a clearly strong-willed woman like her! Her bright eyes of piercing blue glared at me over the top of thick-lensed horn-rimmed spectacles, equalled in impact only by her formidable bosom. This she thrust forward aggressively, defying any mere male to look let alone touch. In addition to the bosom and eyes, the woman possessed a most striking moustache that very few teenage males could hope to equal!

This formidable figure demanded to know who I was and what my business was in her department. Automatically, I sprang to attention and told her. Her booming voice announced that I was late, many minutes late. Ignoring my mumbled excuses about getting lost in the maze of corridors, she continued. "They are waiting for you." Her voice boomed around the still room. I dared not ask who 'they' were. In total silence she ushered me down more corridors deeper into the building, eventually to arrive at a large and ornately-carved pair of double oak doors. She tapped and went in. With a scowl she indicated that I should remain outside. After a few minutes the door opened and with a brief nod of her head, she indicated that I should enter.

With a high degree of trepidation I entered a very large, ornate and dimly illuminated, panelled room. On every wall were huge paintings of very important looking gentlemen in red robes. An enormous oval table of dark oak took up the whole of the floor space. With some difficulty I observed a group of figures seated at one end of the table. The formidable one instructed me to sit at the other end and then to my great relief, swept from the room. The table was so large I could hardly see the group in the gloom.

The interview started at once. Fortunately, I had good hearing and could hear all their questions, but although I spoke up, I felt many of my interviewers could not hear my replies. The sound of gentle snores made it very noticeable that one old lady had gone to sleep. No one seemed inclined to wake her.

Reflecting later, I enjoyed the interview. It was in effect a pleasant chat and soon apparent that apart from the Chairman, a very tall and very distinguished gentleman, no one seemed to know why I was there! I later discovered they were mostly Councillors and that they attended interviews mainly because they enjoyed having a day out in the impressive room. Among the group was one very old man in an ill-fitting navy blue uniform with silver badges on his shoulders and blue oak leaves on the collar. He sat to one side and said nothing at all during the session.

I sailed through the interview and, after putting their heads together and muttering, the Chairman smiled and offered me the job. I delightedly accepted. The distinguished gentleman stood up and, announcing he was the County Medical Officer, asked me to follow him to his office. Once the door was closed behind us the doctor said he would give me a medical there and then. Requesting I strip to the waist, he left the room to attend to another matter.

As I stood waiting for his return, a young lady – this time very attractive – entered with two cups of tea on a tray. I thanked her politely, noticing her dark eyes looking at my half-naked body. At once I had a feeling I was going to enjoy this job! I was certainly ready for the tea, and had almost finished the cup when the doctor returned. He looked a little surprised but said nothing. The medical was very rudimentary; after a few questions and a poke about with a stethoscope (which took him a long time to find) I was pronounced fit. As I was fastening my shirt the old gentleman in uniform entered and was introduced as the Chief Ambulance Officer. I felt myself colour up when the doctor told the Chief he would have to request a new cup of tea! The CAO said very little apart from telling me that I would be appointed, subject to a driving test, stressing it was a police driving test.

I began to feel a little unsure of myself; things were suddenly beginning to get serious.

Having been called to the station and taken the driving test, described previously, I was delighted, after a month, to receive my letter of appointment. Little did I realise that the Ambulance Service at that time had great difficulty recruiting staff for that particular station. Given that I possessed a full quota of limbs, could walk unaided and even do joined-up writing, I was assured of the job!

The letter of appointment contained many details of what to do and what not to do. It was noticeable there seemed to be a lot more 'nots' than 'whats'. Also detailed was a long list of misdemeanours that would result in dismissal. The letter instructed me to report to the Station Officer to arrange a convenient starting date.

I was washed, changed and at the station within half an hour. Full of excitement, I presented myself at the office and immediately discovered I was of less interest to Mr Green as a new staff member than as a potential recruit. I was brusquely told the Station Officer was very busy but his L/A would deal with me in due course.

The L/A, Leading Ambulanceman, or leading hand, demonstrated that he too was just as important as the Station Officer. This was achieved by making me stand in front of the desk and wait whilst he occupied his time with sorting out some very important papers. This task was evidently of great consequence to the well being of the Service, although it seemed to involve nothing more than looking at a paper, grunting, sniffing, then putting it down and looking at another. At no time did he touch a pen or refer to any of the many books or ledgers piled high on his desk. It was clearly an act to impress upon me that the L/A was boss and I was the underdog. Whilst he continued to push papers around his desk in the quest to look important, I was able to study him. He was a man of about sixty, skinny and stooped. Thin straggly white hair fell to the collar of a badly fitting tunic where it rested among dandruff and a layer of dust and grime. The baggy uniform had the look of belonging to one who spent all his days indoors at a desk. The back, elbows and cuffs were shiny, the front a mixture of fag ash, tea stains and embedded grease. The top edge of each breast pocket was emphasised by a ridge of dust. One solitary and faded Defence Medal ribbon indicated his war had not involved him straying far from the station. Granny type gold rimmed specs were perched on the tip of his nose, both lenses thick with grease and fingermarks. The blue shirt collar was too large for his scrawny neck and a paper clip served as a collar stud. He had the unhealthy pallor of someone unaccustomed to fresh air and the lumpy red nose of a boozer, below which was a straggly whisper of a moustache, heavily stained with nicotine. He had the continuing and repellent habit of pushing one corner of this 'tash' into his mouth and noisily sucking. I began to wonder what kind of service I had joined!

At last the Leading Ambulanceman deemed the new recruit had been correctly put in his place and leant back in his chair, placing his hands at the back of his head. It was then I noticed the exceedingly prominent ears. They were unbelievable! I was not at all surprised to learn later that his nickname was 'Noddy'.

In a rasping voice the L/A talked down to me as he did to everyone, unless they were senior, in which case he positively fawned. His language was appalling. It was said that if you stopped him using a certain 'f' word he would become silent! I was soon to discover that Noddy was useless at his job and the butt of many jokes and tricks. We both knew at once we were not going to get on, taking an instant dislike to each other. Whilst he talked, I became aware of the single grubby chrome bar on each shoulder of his uniform, and began to develop aspirations of promotion.

At the end of a long lecture, and after much studying of the duty list and sucking the end of a pencil, the old man told me to report for duty at 0800 hours the following Tuesday morning, St Valentines day. With that the interview was terminated and I went home. Despite meeting Noddy, I was eager to start my new job and become an ambulance-man, a little puzzled though, for I could not get over the fact that I would be on the payroll from Sunday but was to have a rest day on Monday. I didn't understand shifts and couldn't grasp why I needed to rest before I'd done anything! But I didn't mention that to Noddy...

CHAPTER TWO

The First Day

I had great difficulty sleeping the night before I was due to start my first shift, awake longer than asleep, thoughts mixing with dreams. Visions of attractive young ladies in see-through nighties flinging their arms around my neck, merged with horrible nightmares of blood and smashed cars. The boy with the cut head in the park kept appearing in each. At five o'clock I gave up all hope of sleep. Careful not to disturb my sleeping wife, I silently dressed and crept out of the house to take the dog for a walk. The dog, amazed to see anyone up at that hour, leapt out of his basket and wagged his tail.

The town was still and dark and I was surprised at how hushed the streets were at that time of day. It would not to be long before I became only too well acquainted with what it was like to be out and about all night, and to drive through deserted streets, shared only by cats and coppers. The dog and I returned whilst all was still asleep. I was excited and couldn't wait to start my new job. Time dragged slowly until I could report to the station at 0745 hours. The place was already the scene of great activity. Men in navy blue uniforms were busily checking ambulances, topping up oil and water, writing details onto journey records, everyone busy. Everyone seemed to be happy and the air was loud with cheerful banter.

As the new boy, I received a begrudging welcome from Noddy. I later discovered that Mr Green, or 'Godly' as he was generally known, did not like to come into contact with the workers, preferring to arrive later, when everyone had left on their morning runs. Someone said "Godly likes the streets to be aired before he ventures out to start a hard day of doing nothing!"

The L/A stared hard at me over his begrimed specs. It was clear he was not too sure of what to do with me. He had no doubt forgotten about the new boy starting that day. At last, following a violent bout of coughing, which he managed without removing the spindly hand-rolled cigarette from his mouth, Noddy opened the window and loudly shouted across the yard to someone.

"Yoncuminterdeffinofficenarh."

Well at least that's what it sounded like to my untrained ear. I assumed there must be a foreign gentleman working on the station. A moment later the office door crashed open and a red faced, rotund man about my own age stood in the doorway looking at Noddy, an outsize smile creasing his round cheerful face. In his hand he held a pint sized oil can which he offered to the scowling L/A.

"Was you attempting to attract my attention from me duties Mr Blacket, or happen you were having a bilious attack? Mebbe you required me to give you an enema with this pint of Bookum's best to help you manage the day?"

His bright blue eyes twinkled in his chubby red face and the cheery smile became broader.

"If that was your desire, I'd be delighted to oblige you. Or happen you wanted an oil change for your uniform?"

"Yer an effin cheeky young sod Jonesy. Dunno why I puts up wi yer". Noddy gave a deep sniff, noisily cleared his throat and paused to re-light the apology for a cigarette. "Tek this ere new fella away wi yer an show 'im the ropes". He scowled at the other man, who continued to smile broadly. Noddy's lower jaw jutted out in what he presumably took to be a fierce stance. Jonesy beamed even more cheerfully back at him and gave a broad wink.

"Go on Noddy. Giz a kiss!"

With that, he disappeared out of the door before the old man could throw the duty board he was holding at the departing figure. Whilst the L/A grumbled about lowering standards and lack of respect to elders and betters, I quietly slipped out after Jonesy.

Ian Jones bade me welcome to what he described as 'the tattiest station in the county'.

"First thing you gotta learn luv, don't let Noddy or any of them there bastards in yonder get on top of yer. They're all useless. Gi' it back to 'em and they'll back off. If they think you'll kowtow to 'em, they'll never let up."

It took me some little time to discover that most people from that part of South Yorkshire called everyone 'Luv' – even other men! Until I had established this fact, I was a little cautious of Ian.

Again I began to wonder what I'd had joined, but that apart, I felt at once I was going to get on well with Jonesy. He introduced himself and quickly announced that he was from Sheffield. He was broad South Yorkshire in speech and mannerisms and exceedingly proud of it. As we walked across to the vehicle garage, Ian explained that he had been a long-distance lorry driver. He had married a local lass, settled down in the town and joined the Ambulance Service two years previously.

He showed me around the 'bus' we would be using that day. Like most of the fleet it was a large white Bedford J1 ambulance. It looked immaculate and shone like new. I very soon discovered that this was because all staff on the station spent ages, when not on the road, cleaning and polishing the vehicles.

Opening the wide rear doors of the ambulance Ian explained how the stretcher worked, it was a very clever arrangement. The stretcher was an alloy sprung bed with a mattress and raising back rest controlled by a winding handle. A clip allowed the contraption to be slid out of the vehicle by one man until it rested on a tray. His crewmate then slid it to the side, which enabled it to be lifted and carried. I later learned that for heavy or long lifts a thoughtful employer provided canvas straps to go over your shoulders and onto the handles of the stretcher. We moved inside the vehicle where Ian opened and closed numerous lockers, showing where everything was stored. He didn't attempt to explain what the kit was used for, only where it was kept. I thought there seemed to be an awful lot of blankets and triangular bandages, but was soon to learn it was surprising what could be done with both items of equipment.

Glancing at his watch, Ian announced it was time to go. Climbing into the cab he struggled a not inconsiderable belly behind the steering wheel whilst I took the attendant's seat. Reaching across the dashboard Ian picked up the radio and called in to 'Control', telling them we were 'mobile on local duties'. It appeared that the name of the ambulance was 'Sugar'. This seemed a funny name to call an ambulance, but I later discovered that each vehicle had a radio call sign based on the phonetic alphabet, and this was the name by which they were known on the station and to Control.

Twisting the key, Ian started the engine and allowed it a few moments to warm up. As he expertly swung the 'bus' out of the gates, I sat by his side in the attendant's seat feeling very proud. Ian explained that we were on the usual 'milk run' that morning, taking a group of regular patients to the Day Hospital.

With the 'detail sheet' resting on my knee I proudly looked down from my lofty perch at the public as they hurried about their business. I felt very important. I was now a public servant, paid by the ratepayers, there to help them, attend to their every need, ready to go to their aid when required, and give care comfort and support to them in their hour of need. I smiled benevolently whilst looking out of the cab window at those in my care, and they, in return, completely ignored me!

Ian and I got on well and chatted about all sorts of things. I asked when I could drive and was told 'after lunch'. Looking at the large radio with its range of switches and dials, emitting a stream of strange garbled words, I asked whether I could use it. Ian said he would instruct me when Control called. I gazed out of the cab window; everything looked so very different from so high. I was seeing the world from a new viewpoint. I felt very proud and very superior. At last I was doing a worthwhile job. Looking across at my new mate nonchalantly easing the Bedford through the early morning traffic I asked the question uppermost on my mind. 'When could I go to an emergency'. Ian glanced across at me, his round face split into a huge grin.

"When they call us, Luv!"

I frowned, not understanding. Thinking Ian had misheard my question.

"No, what I mean is, when will they send me away for training and then allow me to go to emergencies."

Ian took his eyes off the road for a moment. The shiny round face creased into a wider grin.

"I take it Luv, that Godly Green gave you the same briefing he gave me when I joined?"

I frowned and looked puzzled. This was getting beyond me. The man was talking in riddles.

"I guess he told you sweet FA about us operating procedures?"

I conceded that Godly had not said a lot, apart from what he considered to be the better points of the job. Ian's grin came back.

"As I just said. When they call us, we'll go and do the emergency. Don't worry kid, I'll show thee what to do."

I had sort of assumed that today was just a 'taster' – a chance to see what things were like before I was sent on a training course, like the ones in the Army. I would be taught how to deal with patients and with injures and illnesses that patients suffered. But, Ian quickly made it clear that I had been wrong. Realisation and horror dawned on me slowly, frightening the life out of me. We were to respond and attend whatever incidents occurred within our patch! Ian would deal with the incident whilst instructing me. Instructing me what to do! I was scared. I knew nothing about first aid or anything connected with the subject of injury and illness, nor did I have any idea of how to deal with people in emergency situations. A silly thought sprang to mind, the memory of my first game of snooker. We were playing as a foursome and my partner had remarked he had no chance of winning as he had 'three people playing against him'! I did so hope we didn't get a call and that Ian was better at his job than that snooker player had been!

As I slowly got over the immediate shock and accepted that very soon I was to be facing situations I was not prepared for, Ian explained that, like all the others, I would have to learn as I went along. The news really frightened me. I sat deep in thought, worrying and panicking as we drove around parts of the town I didn't even know existed. At last, Ian pulled up outside a house and told me to go and collect our first outpatient of the morning.

By now I was a bundle of nerves, wondering what to expect. With great trepidation I knocked on the door of the semi-detached house. The front door was opened almost at once and a cheerful tubby woman waddled out, struggling into a fur coat that had seen far better days. The woman stopped, and through ornate diamante-framed glasses, inspected me closely. At last, apparently satisfied, she patted her headscarf covering steel curlers and waddled down the path, chattering non stop until I thankfully closed the back doors on her. The ambulance moved on to our next patient. Very soon the interior was full of patients who all seemed to knew one another. As they were collected each studied me closely, I felt very much the new boy. As each nodded approvingly I began to feel a little more at ease, however, I learnt a first valuable lesson regarding dealing with outpatients when, after saying good morning to an old lady, I foolishly asked how she was. The lady stopped in her tracks.

"Ee lad! Tha's no idea of troubles I've suffered!" She grasped my arm, and as we stood on the path she told me in graphic detail about each of the many health problems she'd suffered since childhood. It took some time to shepherd her into the ambulance. Eventually we arrived at our destination – the Day Hospital. After we had helped everyone into the department and got them settled, Ian led the way and I blindly followed him – into the kitchen for our first cup of tea of the day. This was my second lesson of the day. Never refuse tea... you may not get chance of another one.

The rest of the shift passed in the same fashion: picking up people, taking them to hospital or clinics, and taking others home after treatment. Everyone seemed to know everyone else; they had all been attending for years. Apart from my twitching every time the radio crackled, the day passed well. We did no more than act as transport for outpatients.

I learned a lot from Jonesy that first day. Like most of the other drivers, he had a low opinion of Ambulance Management, especially at our station. Godly Green was next to useless, bluffing his way out of making any decision, especially those that could rebound on him! The two L/As were even worse. Noddy (his name had started as 'Big Ears' moved to 'Noddy's Mate' and then just 'Noddy') attempted to bully anyone foolish enough to allow him to. Most stood up for themselves, so he picked on his colleague, the other L/A. This man was named 'Flapper' Furguson, and was a man who would break into a panic at almost any situation. Both men had been on the Service for donkey's years and had – or so it was said – been promoted into the office because they were useless for any other role. Not for the first time did I began to doubt my wisdom in joining!

In these days before 'stress' had been invented, if you had a job that exposed you to disturbing situations then you just 'got over it like a man.' It was Ian Jones who taught me to look for the funny side of things, something I never forgot for the whole of my service. During that first day Ian related a string of humorous experiences. At the time I thought them to be exaggerated, but very soon found that life in the Ambulance Service was just like that.

At last we returned to the station, washing down the outside and mopping out the inside of the ambulance. I quickly discovered why ambulances always looked so good. Although everyone looked after them, the L/As would insist they were polished, rather than allow anyone to do nothing, even if 'doing nothing' involved reading a first aid book. When all was finished, the two of us stood with the ambulance between us and the office, talking until the clock swung on to six when we could go home. I hadn't done a lot, but was tired, and very proud at the end of my first day as an ambulanceman. I was delighted that we had not covered any emergencies, in fact I was surprised that nobody we had conveyed appeared to really need an ambulance! I left the station that night, proud to feel I belonged. I was also looking forward to tomorrow as Noddy had said they would try to find me a uniform.

CHAPTER THREE

Uniform Issue

Reporting for duty the next day I was very pleased that Ian was to be my mate again. I'd taken to this likeable Yorkshireman, always a cheerful character, always well-liked by patients. Nothing seemed to annoy Ian and he would come back with a joke on every occasion. That man was a good friend to me, especially in those first few days, when he knew I needed to gain the confidence that no officer of the Service had bothered to provide. In addition to a pleasant manner and cheery countenance, Ian was always smart and clean. Unlike most staff members, his uniform fitted well and was pressed and brushed each day. Like most, he wore the metal first aid badge of a voluntary aid society on his left arm, but Ian's, instead of being plain white metal, had been polished until it shone like the proverbial new penny. His shoes were bulled to perfection, the peak of his cap slashed like a guardsman. This, together with the single military General Service Medal stitched above the breast pocket of his tunic, proclaimed Ian was an ex-serviceman. As everyone had to do National Service it was not unusual to be able to pick out one who had 'done his bit' and Ian was obviously proud of his service with the colours. I found he had gained the medal in Malaya and assumed he had been an infantryman. It came as a surprise when, years later, Ian confided that he had served as an Ordinance clerk, well away from any jungle patrols or other distasteful aspects of service life in the Far East.

Again we were allocated to the same 'bus'. 'S' for Sugar was like most of the fleet, a Bedford J1 with an old type coach-built body. The newer vehicles were of a cheaper design and manufacture, and Sugar was accepted as the best vehicle on that Station. The ambulance was allocated to Ian and another guy called Bill. Both men were both fanatical about the old ambulance and were for ever cleaning and polishing. That ambulance was a credit to both builder and Service. I was pleased to be allowed to drive that morning, very well aware I still had a lot to learn about driving a large ambulance, and I was only too conscious of Ian's grimace of pain every time I crunched a gear. I was sure he suffered physical pain when his beloved Sugar was tortured at the hands of one so uncouth. Again we had the 'milk run' of outpatients for the day hospital. I discovered that this was our normal role when on a day shift. Up and down streets, wherever possible picking up and dropping off, always trying to meet the appointment times of patients, although I never quite understood why, as the bookings and office staff never seemed to take such matters into account.

It was mid morning and we'd just taken the main load of patients into the department when we were given an urgent admission. A Miss Chambers was to be in hospital within the hour. I tried to hide my disappointment that it was not an emergency but this was a start. The first non routine patient of my career! With feelings of excitement, I rushed out to the vehicle. Ian followed with little sign of hurry as I sat behind the wheel with engine revving. I didn't dare mention to Ian but the idea of carrying attractive young ladies in flimsy nighties mentioned by Mr Green as a possibility of the job was upper most in my mind. Nothing naughty, but the thought was certainly there. What would Miss Chambers be like? She sounded to be a smasher!

My spirits dropped somewhat as we pulled up outside the dingy terrace house in the poorer part of town. It looked rather old fashioned and faded, not the sort of decor young people chose. Ian climbed out of the cab telling me to follow and do exactly as he told me. The thought of not doing so had never crossed my mind!

A very old lady opened the door and invited us in, ignoring Ian's cheery "Ow do Luv". On rheumaticy old legs she slowly took us upstairs. Everything was dark and dingy; heavy brown paint, dark wallpaper, dim, low-wattage bulbs providing little illumination. At the top of the stairs, we followed the slow old lady into a bedroom. It took some time for my eyes to become accustomed to the light, or rather lack of it, for the room was even darker than the rest of the house. Thick dark curtains were drawn and a single dim light bulb high in the ceiling did little to help us. The room was full of heavy old furniture, every surface covered with ornaments and old photographs. In the centre of a large double bed lay an even older lady, thin as a rail, almost birdlike. From under the wispy grey hair showing below a knitted bonnet, piercing dark eyes flickered between the two of us. She was certainly in a nightie, but this was not quite what I had been hoping for!

The first old lady slowly and carefully explained that her companion on the bed was going into hospital. She firmly stressed many times it was the hospital and not the sanatorium. I would eventually learn all about old people and their preconceived ideas of the hospital system. The patient, who was clearly as deaf as a post, continuously asked why two men where in her bedroom. Ian took control and although she could not hear him, he very quickly had her complete trust.

Ian showed me how to cover the patient in a blanket before removing the bed covers and then how to lift her on to the carry chair. Within a moment our patient was tucked up safe and sound in the blanket and secured to the chair with a broad safety strap. With no effort at all, for she was so small, we carried our patient downstairs in the chair and into the ambulance. It was one of the easiest lifts I was to experience in all my service years. The other old lady donned hat and coat and was helped into the back of the ambulance. My colleague joined them in the back and chattered non stop whilst I found my way to the hospital. More by good luck than judgement I found the right entrance.

By the time our patient was put into bed on the ward, it was lunchtime, when I met my fellow new starter. Ted had started on the same day as me but on a different shift. Although I'd never spoken to him, I had often seen Ted about town for he lived a few streets away from me and had the sort of face you noticed. A very tall and gaunt man, he had a long and pale face with a permanent morose expression above a thick moustache. I was not at all surprised to learn that until the previous week he had been an undertaker! The news that the station now had a butcher (me) and an undertaker (Ted) caused great merriment among our new colleagues!

As I was to quickly learn you can't tell a person's nature from their looks, for Ted was one of the funniest men I was ever to have the good fortune to work with. His sense of humour was as dry as tinder and, as everyone on the station was to find, Ted had a fund of stories, yarns from his wartime service in the Guards and many years as an undertaker. I was soon to discover that to spend a night shift with Ted resulted in sore sides from laughing so much. At the proverbial drop of a hat Ted could tell the most hilarious tales with appropriate facial expressions and actions. Whilst some stretched the bounds of credibility, each was guaranteed to be hilarious.

Ian and I met the other crew as they arrived at the General Hospital. Ted's partner was a man known simply as Alf, a man as short as Ted was tall. As there were no patients ready, the four of us obtained permission from Ambulance Control and went for lunch in the staff canteen. After enjoying a first class meal at a remarkably reasonable cost, we telephoned our station for afternoon duties. Ian and Alf, were instructed to pair up whilst Ted and I were instructed to return to station. Return to be issued with uniform! The Leading hand gave the instruction that the two new boys were to return to the station in the same vehicle with strict instructions for us not to turn on the radio and to keep out of trouble!

Feeling quite proud of ourselves, alone and entrusted with one of the County Council's ambulances, we two new boys cheerfully made our way back to the station and our meeting with the Station Officer. To us Mr Green, the Station Officer, or as we soon discovered, Godly, was a mystic figure, a figure we lesser mortals saw little of. Tom and I had both briefly met the Chief Ambulance Officer but it had been stressed the CAO was far too important to leave headquarters and County Hall. We were to discover that when this apparent demigod did visit our Station, Godly and the Leading Hands panicked and made sure everyone was out or looking busy and polishing things!

Godly Green had been the Station Officer for a good number of years and it was apparent the man considered time was well overdue for him to be promoted to higher things. Like all people in authority in those days Godly was one of the old school with very fixed views. Mr Green considered training to be a waste of time for it prevented ambulancemen polishing things. Polished things were a very important part of Mr Green's working environment. Both Ted and I had noticed the station had the same smell as an Army barracks – Brasso and floor polish. Every light switch and doorknob was made of brass and shone brightly. The office floors were covered in thick brown linoleum, which in turn was covered in an equally thick coating of a red greasy polish. Whilst it smelt nice, we soon discovered that this was all it achieved. Polishing the office floor was a nightly task for the night shift. The established procedure was to toss the stuff down in large globules on top of any dust and dirt, then buff the surface with a heavy duty floor polisher. Everyone failed to understand what this achieved, apart from keeping Godly Green happy. The nickname of 'Godly' had been applied many years before as a result of his favourite expression. 'Cleanliness is next to Godliness.'

Ted and I pulled into the station and duly reported to the station office as requested. Noddy's scowled welcome was most discouraging. He told us Mr Green was a very busy man and we would have to wait.

Ted cheerfully responded, 'OK, we'll go into the rest room'.

At this a look of panic appeared on the old L/A's wrinkled face.

"Yer can't go in there. I've just bulled the floor and Mr Green aint seed it yet".

Ted, a good head taller than the stooped L/A, stepped closer, causing the old man to back away a pace. He scowled down at him. "Well you'll bloody well 'ave to do it again when we've gone, wont you?"

Leaving an angry Noddy blustering and threatening to tell Mr Green about Ted's attitude, we sauntered into the 'rest room', which turned out to be a rather grandiose title for a dull and shabby little room containing a few battered and ancient armchairs and very little else. Within a few minutes Godly stalked in, very full of his own importance. The Station Officer had obviously been told of the new man's insolence. Strutting like a Bantam cock, the piggy eyes flashed behind the pebble lenses of his glasses. But, as the little man squared up to Ted, who rose to his feet and scowled down, Mr Green clearly had second thoughts and chose to ignore the complaint of his subordinate.

"Right-oh men, let us see what we can find to make you look like real ambulancemen. Follow me."

With that, Green marched briskly out of the room, leaving us to follow him across the yard. Despite his immaculate uniform and highly polished shoes, Godly Green was a bit of a joke. At five feet two and fifteen stone, he did not have the figure to look impressive in uniform and certainly not to cut the dash he hoped. He waddled rather than walked across the yard, and I had great trouble holding myself from laughing out loud as Ted imitated the little man's rolling gait behind his broad back.

With the two of us being ex-army, we had expected to be taken to a uniform store and kitted out with everything we needed to at least look the part, even if we didn't know what to do. We were both therefore somewhat surprised to find ourselves taken down the steps into what was obviously the station boiler house. From his trouser pocket Godly produced a large bunch of keys and having ponderously selected the correct one, very carefully unlocked a small rusty tin locker. We looked on in amazement as Green produced a large old canvas sack and began to rummage in it like a small child at Christmas. At last, with a triumphant look on his face like that of a conjurer, he pulled a dusty second-hand cap out of the sack with a flourish. He peered at each of us intently and then held it out to Ted. "Try that". The cap fell over Ted's ears covering his eyes. Godly's piggy eyes glinted through the thick glasses. "Perfect, put a bit of newspaper in the sweat band."

He proceeded to pull out further creased and dusty items of uniform. Obviously, when anyone left the Service they handed in their uniforms. These were kept and issued to new starters until they received a new consignment. Most of the contents of the sack looked as though they had been in there for donkey's years, each item covered in mildew and dirt. Ted found a cap that fitted better than the first but with no badge. I received a pair of black shoes covered with green mould. We thanked Godly, but declined to accept either. The little Station Officer seemed to be very put out, as though the starving were refusing food. We were both convinced the man took a dislike to the pair of us from that day, never forgiving us for spurning his efforts.

Ted and I waited something like six months for the issue of our uniforms. The other staff assured us that our uniforms would arrive by then, for after seven months the Council was required to pay us two shillings (10p) a week 'uniform allowance'. I spent the ensuing period wearing a navy blue suit with Ted looking even less like an ambulanceman in a brown sports coat!

CHAPTER FOUR

Plug in the Standby Crew

I remember staring in bewilderment at the impressive item of furniture. A masterpiece of long lost craftsmanship, deep red mahogany, the surface polished and glowing with the patina of age. Along the front was a row of silver eyeballs, each with a painted number, these dropped with a frightening buzz when activated. Brass plugs like rows of knitting needles, or perhaps bullets, stood protecting the front of the 'thing' against attack. These plugs were in turn attached by long corded leads to the innards of the 'thing'. It was a work of art, a masterpiece, a telephone exchange built to contain every item of modern technology known to man at the turn of the twentieth century. If it still existed it would be worth a fortune. But, no doubt it would have been thrown away years ago.

Having spent a week on days learning the ropes, or at least what a rope was, and where they were kept, I was now about to start my first night shift. Having just begun to get used the idea of the job I discovered myself due to work a period of nights. Apart from army guard duty I'd never been up all night before!

The shift pattern was midnight to eight and I'd had the previous day off as a rest day. But of course, I'd got up to help get my son off to school, then taken the dog out and helped about the house, doing nothing in particular, just waiting to go to work. As a result of my activities, by 11pm I was more ready for bed than a night shift. My wife retired whilst I sat twiddling my fingers waiting for the clock to reach eleven forty-five. By the time it did I was worn out.

I cycled the short distance down to the station arriving at the same time as Bill, my mate for the night. Entering the office we prepared to take over from the back shift crew, who were naturally keen to go home. I had not met any of these men before. Smithy was a smallish man with a luxurious set of carefully tended whiskers. I'd heard of him and had been told he was always cheerful and joking, at his happiest when imitating Godly Green. Most people said Smithy was more true to form than the man himself! Smithy's mate that evening was Jack, seemingly ancient and very near to retiring age. With our entry Smithy leapt to his feet.

"Come on you Jack, old fool, I told your missus I'd get you home early tonight in case she's feeling a bit frisky."

Jack, who was noted for being continually cantankerous, miserable, and poor company, scowled and grumbled.

"Bog orf 'miffy. You wait till you get to my age, and you'll be pleased to get to bed to sleep."

With this banter continuing non-stop these two ill-matched characters gathered their kit and wasted no time in bidding us goodnight.

I had never met Bill before but had been pleased to be told he would look after me. I most certainly needed someone to do this! Bill looked to be a very old man. His thin, gaunt face was lined and weather-beaten; he was tall and exceedingly thin, his shoulders rounded, causing him to stand and walk with a permanent stoop. I was to discover that although only in his mid thirties, Bill liked to give the impression of being far older and mature. It was also clear that Bill had a quiet air of efficiency about him, a manner that gave confidence to all his patients. It certainly gave confidence to me! Bill solemnly shook hands and introduced himself, and while doing so, switched on the kettle. Removing his uniform cap he exposed a prematurely bald head, which greatly added to his elderly looks. He announced importantly he would telephone Control, tell them that we were on duty and then show me the routine of night shift. Following him through the hallowed portals of the Leading Hand's office, my eyes wandered over the general untidiness of the room. An array of dusty uniforms hung from wall pegs, bits of ambulance equipment covered every surface, piles of yellowing paper and much-thumbed record books. Bundles of daily worksheets tied with string, an array of battered and chipped mugs and cups (apparently no two alike)

Then I saw the 'thing' for the first time. Bill crossed to it and turned to beam at me. Turning back, my new colleague looked at it proudly and rubbed the polished wood with the cuff of his tunic.

"Beautiful workmanship! You couldn't get wood like that nowadays if you paid a king's ransom!"

Bill picked up the handset in one hand and a brass plug in the other. Carefully lifting the plug to his lips he took a deep breath and huffed onto it, then slowly and lovingly polished the brass against the cuff of his jacket. When apparently satisfied he slid it gently into a hole on the front of the 'thing' and flicked a brass switch a number of times. After a few minutes wait, whilst Bill alternated between polishing the wood with the tunic cuff and wiping each of the other brass plugs against the leg of his trousers, he started to speak. After enquiring after the health of the other person, the weather, moaning about the lack of success with the national pay talks, he proceeded into a lengthy discussion about rabbits, although it was only after several minutes conversation that I discovered it was about rabbits, for he talked about 'lops'.

As Bill talked, I made tea. I knew little about the job, but knew the important thing was to get a cuppa whenever you could. Whilst Bill continued his conversation, he went into sign language and a set of facial expressions to indicate he wanted tea strong and sweet. Bill took the offered mug and continued with his conversation. By this time he seemed to be deeply engrossed into the sex life of lops.

At last, after arranging to meet the voice at the other end of the line at a local rabbit show at the weekend, Bill put down the handset and beamed at me over the rim of his mug.

"You've joined us at a very important and sad time lad. A moment of 'istory you'll be able to tell your grandchildren about. Thee and me do three nights and when we come here again this beauty will be gorn…" Bill started to polish the wood again with the cuff of his tunic. I am sure there was the hint of a tear in his eye. "…gorn for ever, and, we'll 'ave been *modernised*."

He went on to explain that by then all emergency calls would go through to Control ("who don't know what they are doing most of the time - as fik as two short planks wi' out nails") It would then be their job to ring us and give us the details.

"But," he continued, "at present, when the public rings 999, that there red eyeball will drop and the buzzer will go. We takes the job and go orf ter do it. But, 'afore we go, we plug in the standby crew, then the next call will go through to them in bed. They'll come un get an ambulance and go and do the job. When we get back we take over again." He very obviously preferred things to remain as they were. As the new boy I wondered what happened if a third call came through whilst we were all out, but in Bill's sentimental mood it seemed churlish to ask.

We went out to the garage to check the ambulance. The night was bitterly cold and Bill raided two other vehicles, collected their hot water bottles, filled each with boiling water and put them between our blankets. When all was done to his satisfaction we went back into the warmth of the office.

Those first two hours rushed by as we did other routine chores. As we worked Bill told me a lot about the Service once he had accepted the disappointment of me not being a lop lover. He was an ambulanceman of the old school, a man who could not be ruffled. Bill taught me that, although there was not much we could do as ambulancemen, the patient was the most important thing, the only reason for us being there. Nothing caused him to panic, nor would he be rushed. Bill was on top of his job. He was also a good teacher and knew how to explain things so even I could understand.

We sat in two battered arm chairs in front of the smoky old coke stove in the inner office and drank endless mugs of tea as we talked... well Bill talked, I listened. At about three o'clock Bill suddenly went to sleep. My busy day and the warmth of the office was beginning to affect me as well. I was finding it hard to keep awake yet frightened to nod off in case I missed anything.

I must have fallen asleep, because when the buzzer sounded I woke with a fright. Bill was awake, talking into the phone whilst fastening his collar stud with the other hand. Meanwhile, I was trying to work out if I was asleep or awake. We'd got a job.

"Start up lad we've got a 'matty'. I'll plug in the standby crew."

I was out the office and into the ambulance like a jackrabbit. As the engine roared into life I switched on lights and beacons. I was about to go on an emergency! Off to serve my public – deliver a baby. My heart pounded as the adrenaline surged through me. Bill, wrapping a red wool scarf around his neck, unhurriedly opened the double doors of the station. He waited until I had done a racing start out of the station, shut the double doors behind us and climbed into the cab. I was about to let out the clutch when he spoke. "Afore you go son, don't you think it's a bit nippy to be going out in just your shirt?" Feeling a clot I slunk back to the office for my jacket and coat.

Bill let me have my head as we thundered through the deserted streets to the address. As we turned the corner into the street of the call, Bill disappointed me by reaching across and switching off the beacon.

"If she thinks it's that important lad she might 'ave it.... And, I've not had me grub yet!"

The good lady was waiting at her front door and walked out to us. An overcoat on top of her nightie, a headscarf hiding fearsome metal curlers. Our patient climbed into the back of the ambulance and sat chatting non stop to Bill whilst I drove to the hospital. I was rather upset that she didn't have the baby for my benefit!

Bill collected a wheelchair from the porch and together we took the lady to the maternity ward and handed her over to the care of the ward staff. I obediently followed Bill into the kitchen where a nurse responded to his line of chat and made a pot of tea from the ever boiling kettle on the range. Whilst Bill was talking to her, another nurse appeared at the kitchen door and beckoned to me. Putting down my tea mug I of course dutifully followed her to the ward. Giving me a big smile the nurse told me to sit by the door saying "I'll fetch you in when she's ready." I duly sat down as instructed, thinking it was part of the admission system.

I'd been sitting there alone for about five minutes. Reading posters urging me to have my baby injected with all sorts of things and idly skimming through tattered old magazines, when Bill wandered up. "What's up lad? Why yer hiding from me? Have I said summat wrong?"

Before I could respond, the nurse returned and with a big smile announced, "You can come and see your wife now Sir."

Bill burst out laughing, and after a moment the nurse joined him. I looked from one to the other in amazement. It took a moment or two for the penny to drop. Dressed in a blue suit the nurse had taken me for the expectant father – I definitely needed my uniform!

CHAPTER FIVE

Sex and escorts

It was at about this point in my career that I learned about sex. Well it would perhaps be more accurate to say I discovered that patients didn't have sex. Of course when I say they didn't have sex, what I really mean is that the booking system rendered them sexless.

Each morning before commencing the run we would get a list of patient's names, and destinations. These then had to be placed in a running order, with times recorded by us when we picked up and dropped off each patient. The details came from the hospitals and one of the leading hands, or in very rare cases, Godly Green, would write them on to the Service transport forms.

We were absolutely convinced that the two deadbeats were so old they had never been to school. The writing of each was appalling, almost as though a spider had crawled into an ink well and dragged itself across the paper. Many a time I had to go into the office and ask what the word was. I could well imagine Oliver Twist got a better reception asking for extra food than I did asking for clarification. Flapper would take my request as a personal insult. He would start to shuffle his feet, almost running on the spot. His florid face would twitch, whilst one eye would wink grotesquely, the other would look to heaven for inspiration. All the time his knarled old hands would wring in anguish. I was sure that one day Flapper Furguson would burst into tears and sob all over me. Eventually, after this full performance of deep anguish the man would at last quieten down and answer my query. With that he was clearly pleased to get rid of you. But not Noddy...

Noddy was without doubt the most objectionable man I had ever met. Totally useless at his job the old L/A would bluster and shout, but always making sure to evade the problem in hand. We all knew that if in doubt Noddy would rush off to whine to Godly. The Station Officer would in turn nod, make soothing noises, look as though he was going to do something but do absolutely nothing. Noddy's handwriting was unbelievable, worst than any small child. Most staff on the station would recognise the odd word and guess the rest. As the new guy I had no chance.

Noddy would stare at me through the dirty, smoky lenses of his glasses. The bloodshot, bulging eyes would blaze. That outsize bulbous nose would glow, his face would turn a dull shade of red. I always had a horror that Noddy would get so worked up he would collapse with a stroke, leaving me with the nightmare of having to do mouth-to-mouth on him. Even to this day I doubt if I could have done it, and I have dealt with some rough 'uns in my time! Noddy would snatch the offending document from my hands and holding it close to his face stare at it. I was convinced he had difficulty reading the details himself! He would then scowl his best scowl at me. Placing the paper on the desk he would jab at it with a dirty and much chewed fingernail. With each jab the L/A would shout the details at me, each word interspersed with an obscenity.

"If yer 'ad any effin sense yer would sees 'er effin name is effin Miff, Missus effin Miff. Uv effin 'igh Street, ter yer orspital art patients. Fur effin ten er clock"

As this performance was enacted Noddy would blow foul breath and fag ash in my direction. As I retreated from this, he would advance giving me the full benefit of last night's curry and best bitter beer. As recorded I never ever got on with that bloke.

It was on one of the fortunately very occasional days when we were having an enforced few hours together in the office. Noddy was expounding on how good the job had been in the old days. The days before they started to employ 'nancy boys'. And, heaven help the job if they ever let women in! It would be nappies and make-up in the ambulances, and them always going off to have babies or woman's problems every few days.

"Ah tells yer now, young fella, my mussus 'ud create 'ell if any uv um tried ter ger orf wiv me!"

The thought was frightening. Could any woman possibly fancy Noddy! It was these comments about women that prompted me to ask why patients were sexless. The man stared at me in amazement. His mouth dropped open, he started to drool. I learned what a dirty old man looked like!

"They aint" He announced. "Gor blimey, stroof. Nar I cud tells yer a fing or two abart wimmin in the ambulances. I remembers the time..." Noddy then rambled on about some old biddy who had taken a shine to him. I found this very hard to believe. How could it possibly be true? And, he never mentioned even once that she was blind!

I at last managed to ask my question. Why didn't we find out if patients were male or female. Annoyed that I had interrupted his reminiscing, Noddy snapped that it didn't matter. He then muttered that as bookings worked their way around doctor's surgeries, hospital departments, Ambulance Control and to the station, minor details got lost. I didn't see the point but saw no merit in arguing.

The sexless bit was a prime example of how we got stuck with Mrs Bloggs. Like most things it was Smithy's fault, although he denied it, but I expect it could have happened to anyone. Smithy and his mate were on a local outpatient run and had a new regular patient one day. They knocked at the door and after a while an old chap came out buttoning his overcoat against the wind. He nodded back toward the house. "The missus is inside, she'll need an 'and." So the crew went into the house to look for her.

Mrs Bloggs was a lump. There was no more apt description. The lady was about fifteen stone and four foot six, and we had to guess that bit for she never stood up on her feet. She was a handicapped good natured lump, always cheerful and happy, but she could not do a thing for herself. On the other hand her old man was a miserable old so and so, always moaning. The ticket said it was a mister and the patient could walk but no one attached a lot of faith to that. So, the crew fetched their chair from the ambulance, loaded Mrs Bloggs on to it and pushed the lady to the bus.

An ambulance carrychair is a great piece of kit, collapsing away when not required it folds into a handy little chair with wheels to move a patient when needed. Mrs Bloggs was placed on the chair and sort of covered it with her body and a magnitude of scarves and heavy coat. The patient was carefully wheeled to the vehicle and lifted into the back. An ambulanceman very quickly learns how to lift, like most things there is a 'knack' to it. But Mrs Bloggs proved the point that there is an exception to every rule. Whilst she was being loaded, Mr Bloggs sat in the bus and complained about the draught!

Mr and Mrs Bloggs joined our regular patients, everyone groaned if you got their detail, but she was a nice old dear and perhaps the treatment would get her on her feet again soon. The real problem was Bloggs, he was a typical moaner, nothing could suit him. Bloggs moaned from the time of collection until the time he was dropped off, and all the time his wife would be as cheerful as could be.

We all grumbled to Godly and the L/As about the problem but of course they did nothing about it. One or two of us had a moan at the hospital, but that was a waste of time as well. So three times a week someone would be lumbered with carting Mrs Bloggs and the miserable old so and so from their house to the ambulance, ambulance to hospital and then the same in reverse. As we all agreed, she was a lump but a nice old dear, but Bloggs was a pain!

It was the old man's constant complaining about everything, but in the main the draught, as the big rear doors were left open whilst we struggled with his wife, that brought thing to a head one morning. The crew had just battled to get her back into the house after treatment. Old Bloggs stood at his front door moaning as usual about all his 'eat escaping and the fact that we were costing him a fortune in 'lectric bills'. Smithy decided he'd had enough. After helping his mate settle the old lady into her chair he then gently steered the grumpy old man into the other room.

"Mr Bloggs, I don't wish to sound unpleasant, or to appear anti-social, but as you always complain about the cold, or the delays, why don't you stop at home and wait for us to fetch the missus home? You could keep warm in front of the fire and have a nice cup of tea ready for the good lady when we get her back. Now don't you think that would be a good idea?"

The old chap looked at Smithy for some seconds, a pitying look on his lined face. At last he spoke.

"Naw, don't be daft, I gorra go."

Smithy smiled at him. When Smithy smiled, his eyes would crinkle and his beard would stand out. He looked just like a happy gnome. Someone said that if Smithy sat on a toadstool in a garden centre someone would buy him. Smithy's smile said 'I'm a nice guy, I'm here to help so don't sod me about.' It was his special smile, the smile he used on drunks, coppers and other trouble makers.

"Now come along boss, you've got to admit we look after the good lady very well, Mrs Bloggs knows us, and we'll make sure she comes to no harm, won't we?"

The little man stared hard at Smithy.

"Naw I gorra go. I can't miss. Yer sees I need the treatment fur me back."

Smithy stared hard at him, not understanding.

"Do you mean you *both* have treatment then?" he asked rather incredulously.

"Naw, only me... The missus only comes 'cos she enjoys the ride!"

CHAPTER SIX

Blooded

After a few short weeks, I found I was beginning to fit into the pattern of work as an ambulanceman and enjoy the job. For the first time in many years I felt part of an organisation. I still had little idea of what I should or shouldn't do regarding treatment of patients, but I was learning fast. It was very much a case of relying on my mate of the day to look after both me and the patients. I attended incidents and transported patients, found my way around the town and the surrounding area. We visited hospitals and clinics I had never heard of, all in my home town, which I thought I knew well.

I got to know my colleagues, and quickly discovered their foibles and their good and bad points. I also quickly learnt who was good at the job and who was not, who I felt safe with and who I didn't! Their performance on the road apart, I found that the station was more or less evenly divided between the good guys and the toadies. There were some who seemed to delight in passing gossip to the Leading Hands, and anything the L/As learned went directly to Godly.

Godly Green was like nobody I had ever experienced before. He never did a thing about anything. He collected information and stored it like a sponge, some said he had a large book in which he recorded every bad thing he heard about each member of staff, a black list. Godly would arrive each morning at nine fifteen in a shiny little old Austin car, which would be parked directly outside the office door. I never understood if this was to save him walking an extra few steps or to make it difficult for us to get into the office. He would struggle to climb out of the car, open the rear door and very carefully put on his cap. When he was happy that it was correctly fitted, he would remove his briefcase from the back seat, and with great care lock each door of his car. When he was sure it was safe, Green would waddle into the office, and should any of us lesser mortals be within sight, he would pointedly ignore us.

As a rule, we would all be mobile long before he arrived, but on the odd occasion we were in, it would be a treat to watch the daily morning performance. It would start at about five to nine. The duty L/A would suddenly start to rush around, to empty wastepaper baskets, polish the desk and hide things. The strip of carpet would be shaken outside the door and when he was satisfied that all looked right for his lord and master, he would make tea. We used a selection of chipped and cracked cups and mugs scrounged from an array of sources, but Godly Green had his own cup and saucer. Actually, he had two, the second was saved for the odd occasion when the Chief visited the station.

Mr Green's ceremonial daily arrival took the form of a bowing and scraping L/A with a cup of tea. He would take it as though accepting the freedom of the ambulance station, then waddle into his inner sanctum where he would sit in grand isolation for the whole of the day. At four thirty, the process would be reversed and he would waddle out of his office, unlock the car, place his briefcase on the back seat, remove his cap and place it carefully on the seat beside his and then drive off. Mr Green always dressed immaculately and spent his time trying to look important. We never knew what he did in his office during the day. On the odd occasion when he was faced with a problem, he would listen most reluctantly and then make his standard statement, "Leave it with me". Everyone knew that meant that nothing would ever be done about it.

The two old Leading Hands were scared stiff of him. They were like Tweedle Dum and Tweedle Dee. Noddy would spend his days striving to be unpleasant to everyone, and generally succeeding. He blustered his way through life, bullying, whining or hiding from those he feared, furthermore, his personal cleanliness left a great deal to be desired. It was rumoured his uniform stood by itself in a corner when he went to bed at night, it was so thick with grease. His writing had to be seen to be believed, it was appalling, a child of five could do better. However these many faults faded to insignificance when compared to his language which was the worst I have ever heard. I, like most, had been in the army, but at times cringed at Noddy's limited, repetitive and obscene vocabulary. His priorities appeared to be split between getting to the pub each night and ensuring he was never to blame if anything went wrong.

His colleague was not a lot better. Flapper Furgerson was basically a nice old man, at least he was clean and reasonably smart. He was only months off retirement and for the past few years had believed in taking the easy way out of any problem. Flapper was sometimes known as 'Lightning' – because he always took the easiest route. He had started his working life as a Fireman, and had moved to ambulance duties before the war. On the odd occasion that you could get him to relax and talk, he would relate fascinating incidents of duties in an ambulance during the war – he had served in many parts of the country and had been sent to London at the height of the blitz. It was a great shame that somewhere along the way he had had the stuffing knocked out of him and had retreated into a soft shell. Flapper was now a liability even in the office.

Flapper's nickname had developed by his inborn ability to panic at anything at all. How he coped with fire fighting was a mystery, his panicking was probably why he had been booted out to be an ambulanceman. Whenever the emergency phone rang he would start to panic, the colour would drain from his face, he would stutter and his left eye would twitch alarmingly. Flapper's writing was poor at the best of times but an emergency ticket from him was unreadable. I always had visions of him turning out to an accident by running down the road without an ambulance but with the telephone still in his hand. Sometime I must relate the tale of when he left his mate at the scene of an accident!

As for the hierarchy, I had seen the Chief Officer at my interview and was told he never left Headquarters apart from going to County Hall. I understood there was a Deputy and other officers, but we never saw them. The

L/As said they had very important things to do at Headquarters, something that didn't bother us at all. We were not at all sorry they never came to see us. Looking back to those far off days, I am amazed that the service functioned at all. It seemed that most ambulancemen tried hard to provide a service to the patients in spite of, rather than because of, the system! There was little equipment, no training and an awful amount of guesswork. There was also a small element of staff who got by doing little or nothing at all.

Promotion was based on age, ability having nothing to do with it, and man-management was something totally unheard of.

Somehow we managed, and whilst the standards were lacking through no fault of the staff, patient care was based on dedication and was of a high standard. It was widely reported, and I imagine very accurately, that the Chief Ambulance Officer had once stated, "Don't increase pay or we'll get the wrong sort of chap!" In those days it was a male-dominated service, as it was to remain for some years before any ladies joined us.

I, for one, felt that I was 'the right sort of chap' and enjoyed the life. I was looking forward to getting my uniform to make me feel more a part of it, besides which it was becoming embarrassing being mistaken for a visitor or a patient when I went on to a hospital ward. Furthermore, doctors at patient's houses did not seem to believe me when I said I was an ambulanceman, and on more than one occasion I had to point to the vehicle outside before they were convinced. And it was downright dangerous to be called to a punch up in a pub or dance hall.

I had only been on the job a few weeks when I discovered that people were beginning to recognise me. At the main hospital, the A&E department and outpatient department were linked by a long corridor. During the day it was normally full of patients waiting at their respective department, often overflowing from the waiting area. Walking between the two one morning, seeking my patients, I noticed a young man, and each time I passed he would nod to me. I've never been any good with names but have always remembered faces, but, try as I could, this one was beyond me. At long last curiosity got the better of me and I asked if I knew him. The chap seemed delighted I had spoken to him and smiling broadly proudly replied. "I saw you at the accident you attended last month on the corner of the High Street by the King's Head." I had been to so few accidents that I well remembered the job. I beamed, delighted to have been recognised by a grateful patient.

"Nice to see you, are you getting better?"

The smile faded. "Oh no, I wasn't the patient. I was in the crowd watching!"

The procedure for covering emergencies entailed the nearest ambulance to the scene being re-directed, there were no such luxuries as dedicated emergency crews trained and waiting. If you had patients on board you dropped them at a hospital, or took them home, whichever the quicker. Some quirk of fate had decreed that Ted, who had joined the same day as I, had attended far more emergencies than I. Ted had also covered some bad cases. He had delivered babies, attended fatal accidents, you name it, he went there. Me? I didn't go to anything of interest. When I was on duty, it all stopped. If I was called to a maternity case, she had either given birth before I arrived, or did so two days later; then there was the accident where the casualty had got up and walked back into the pub, or the RTA (Road traffic Accident) where no one was injured. I began to think I would never be called upon to use the skills I had read about in my first aid book.

But like all things in life, everything changes. For me this change came with a vengeance one sunny Sunday morning in June. I was on station with Bob, a very experienced and unflappable ambulanceman when the control phone announced an RTA in the Market Place. Within a few minutes I was to experience what the real world of being an ambulanceman was all about. We pulled up at the scene where the usual crowd had gathered, but they were silent. I soon saw why. A three ton truck had reversed over an eight-year-old boy. I will not attempt to describe his condition. He was still alive – just – but nothing could have saved him. We managed to get him to the hospital only to watch him die in the casualty department. We returned to our vehicle and drove back to the station in silence. Although Bob offered to do it, I forced myself to go into the back of the ambulance and clean up. It was my job as attendant and I knew I had to do it. Fortunately, the rest of the shift involved nothing more than routine admissions. I didn't eat my sandwiches. I'd never felt so low, but it was a feeling I was going to have to learn to live with for the rest of my career as an ambulanceman.

I went home in a very confused and shocked state. My wife knew I had experienced something bad and wisely left me to my thoughts. It was something I had to sort out for myself. I could not stop thinking about my own three year old son. I was in two minds whether to give up the job. Could I take any more incidents like that? I was well aware I was not good company and found sleep would not come that night. I tossed and turned and was out of the house before dawn, needing to be alone with my thoughts. Luckily for me, I didn't get another bad job like that before I was able to come to terms with myself and the realities of the job.

My shock was not helped the following evening when glancing through the local paper and reading the report of the accident. I remember staring at the page in disbelief as it slowly dawned on me that the child involved in the accident was the same child I had picked up from under the climbing frame in the park all those months ago, the accident that had made me decide to join the Service.

CHAPTER SEVEN

Mental Patients

"You're kidding me, aren't you? You're pulling my leg? Go on say you are".

Syd shook his head, "Nope, that's what the man said, that's the job we've got."

I had a horrible feeling in the pit of my stomach. This time I knew my pear-shaped shift mate was not joking. We had been detailed to transport my first mental patient to the County mental hospital.

In those days society understood far less about mental illness than it does today, and it appeared that it had no wish to understand. If you suffered from mental illness the response was to lock you away. Mental illness is far better understood today, people accepting that others can have mental problems just as well as physical illness. Treatment, drugs and attitudes have changed tremendously over the years, but in the 1960s, the subject was not even mentioned. Mental hospitals were unspeakable places, tucked out of sight, hidden from the view of the general public, suffering a stigma similar to that of the workhouse, indeed that was how most had originally been. The few mental hospitals I saw were large rambling Victorian buildings, set well back in their own large grounds, behind high walls and locked gates, hidden from view, out of sight, out of mind. In my own mind, in common with most people, the very term mental patient conjured up visions of the stark raving mad characters portrayed in horror stories. Whilst the subject was never discussed, it was one the public both feared and ignored. I, for one, was scared stiff!

We tided up and moved the ambulance from the garage, well aware it would take a good three hours to do the round trip, we would not be doing any other jobs that shift. During the journey to collect the patient I was in a state of great agitation, wishing I was anywhere other than in an ambulance going to transport somebody to mental hospital. The hospital which served our patch was outside the County Town, some 45 miles away. As Syd was the driver, it was to be my job to travel in the back with the patient. I would much rather have been the driver, but I dare not ask.

We arrived at the address, a large and pleasant house in the 'posh' part of town. Climbing from the bus we were met by the Mental Welfare Officer. He knew Syd, indeed he knew all ambulancemen – apart from me. As I was to learn, the MWO would always meet us at the ambulance, out of sight of the patient and relatives. It was always the same in such cases, a huddled conversation would take place with the MWO giving us details and the required documentation. After a general chat between him and Syd, the MWO told us the gentleman we were to take was a very well-known local figure, a retired solicitor and Alderman. The patient had been sedated and would be no trouble. I didn't believe him! I watched as Syd carefully reversed up the gravel drive to the front door.

I followed Syd and the MWO inside the impressive house, the hall was large enough to drive the ambulance into! Our shoes disappeared into carpet. After climbing a magnificent sweeping staircase we were shown into a very large and grand bedroom. In the centre of a large double bed lay a very old, very fragile, tiny figure, he was so small and frail he hardly made an impression on the upper sheets. I certainly did not recognise him as the impressive and powerful man who had dominated the local scene for so many years. Our patient was fast asleep. After a few more months service, I would be able to recognise that the old chap was senile, and following the well worn path of so many of his generation, being shunted off to a mental hospital, to be out of sight and, excuse the pun, out of mind. But I did not have the required amount of service, nor experience of life to know this. I was very much on edge.

We carefully wrapped the sleeping patient in a blanket and lifted him onto our carrychair. We carried him down the stairs and out to the ambulance. He was so light we could hardy feel him. A number of his relatives gathered at the bottom of the stairs, I didn't realise then that those tears, as they watched us tuck him up on the stretcher, were of the crocodile variety. As the doors closed the group waved him goodbye. Syd gently pulled away and with tyres crunching on the long gravel drive our lengthy journey began. The old man slept peacefully. I should have realised he would be no trouble, and Syd should have told me it was a geriatric case rather than a violent mental patient, but Syd was enjoying his bit of fun at the expense of the new boy. The old man slept like a baby for the whole of the journey and my confidence had almost returned by the time we drove through the gates of the hospital.

The sprawling grey stone buildings of 'St Someone's' hospital, but still referred to as the County Asylum, was a large, impressive and also forbidding establishment. We drove through the high, ornate iron gates and down an immaculate drive which ran between close-cropped lawns and large mature oak trees. At last we came to the hospital. This was an enormous main building with what appeared to be miles of wings going from it in all directions. I was pleased Syd knew the layout and which entrance we needed to be at.

It was then that it suddenly dawned upon me, the place was deserted. It was about eight thirty with darkness fast approaching, yet although each window blazed with light we saw no one through the windows, nor indeed in the grounds. It was an extraordinarily uncomfortable feeling of loneliness, strange and very still, like something from a film. My newly found confidence disappeared. After what seemed an age we arrived at the entrance to the ward. Syd backed the ambulance up to the door, climbed out, walked over to the door and knocked. Pleased we had arrived, even though still very unsure of my surroundings and as my patient was still sleeping his drugged sleep, I climbed out to join Syd. It was silent as the grave, a deadly silence broken only by the sound of the engine ticking as it cooled. Syd banged again on the heavy door again, the sound boomed and echoed, just like the movies… horror movies!

I found myself experiencing rising panic. At last, footsteps could be heard approaching and with much rattling of keys, the door slowly opened, hinges squealing in protest.

The male nurse was a big and burly man, dressed in a short white coat buttoned to the throat. In response to Syd's cheery greeting the man grunted and asked if we got the necessary papers for admission. Syd passed the MWO's bundle to him and we stood in silence whilst the man studied each paper in turn. We were not going to get in unless all was in order. Having checked all to his satisfaction, the nurse invited us to bring in the patient. We off loaded the stretcher and carried it and the patient into the building, waiting whilst the nurse locked the heavy door behind us, we then followed him down a long, brightly lit corridor. The corridor was painted dark brown and cream, the floor covered in highly polished brown linoleum. Apart from the echoing of our footsteps, all was silent and unreal. At long last our escort unlocked another door and we entered the ward. The sight has never left me. Under the high vaulted ceiling, rows and rows of beds, as far as we could see, each containing a still sleeping form. There must have been 100 men in that room, each in bed, each bed in a row, each row in perfect order and each with an identical bedspread. Everyone was asleep!

Two more male nurses were waiting, each large and well built like the first. We followed them to a empty bed at the end of a row and gently lifted our still sleeping patient into it. The first nurse and a colleague very quickly and expertly tucked the blanket and bedspread around the still form. In moments the once important and powerful

Alderman was tucked up as neatly as the others in that silent place. Our peacefully sleeping charge had now become a hospital patient. I often wondered what the man, who had once been so powerful, must have thought when he woke up and found himself in that situation.

We stopped for the inevitable cup of tea and I discovered the nurses were quite normal and friendly men. Nevertheless, I breathed a sigh of relief when we returned to the bus and drove out of the grounds of that huge silent establishment and returned to our home station.

CHAPTER EIGHT

Jack's Tea

I looked in amazement at the Leading Hand.

"You're having me on, aren't you?" I had no faith in Noddy's managerial ability. As an ex-soldier I considered they had given him a rank bar and the title of Leading Ambulanceman, because he was too old and useless for any other role. It stood out a mile, he couldn't lead a horse to water; I did however concede that the expression about organising things in breweries may not apply, for he generally smelt like one in the mornings!

There must have been something in it, some slight grain of truth though, for Noddy stared hard at me without backing off. His watery old eyes glowered behind the dirty glasses. Noddy took the hand rolled apology of a cigarette out from under his straggly nicotine stained 'tash, where it normally lurked, and coughed. I smartly stepped out of his line of fire.

"Am tellin yer, there sendin' yer orf ter 'ospital ter learn yer job." He turned back to his paper strewn desk mumbling about damn young whippersnappers, finking they noes it all. Suddenly he spun around to me angrily, jabbing his finger at me, "When I started on this effin job..."

To catcalls, jeers and a line from 'Tell me the old old story', Ian and I shot out of the office leaving Noddy in full flight.

I had been in the Service almost six months. My training had been what the other lads had taught me, bitter experience gained whilst trying to do my best, leaving me woefully aware of my lack of skills when helping my patients. I now knew from experience that if a patient yelped when I did something, then I must never do that again with that type of injury! I had organised a place on a first aid course with the local Voluntary Aid Organisation and was due to start the weekly two hours per night in a few weeks. Whilst hoping I would learn something, I had to confess the main interest was that it also gained me an extra seven shillings in my weekly pay packet! I looked across at Ian, my mate, my mentor and protector, the fount of all knowledge at the station. "Could the old fool have got something right for once?" Ian shrugged his shoulders and pulled a face. "They've been talking about it for a couple of years now, but they were talking about it when I joined, they always talk. But when it comes to spending money though they change their minds. I shouldn't get too excited about it mate." I sat looking out of the cab window at the passing streets, deep in thought, could it be that for once I was going to be taught something of value? I did so hope it was true.

I had heard the rumour that some lucky staff were to be sent to the General Hospital near Headquarters. They were to spend time in casualty and theatre, to gain knowledge and learn how to give better patient care. Management had indicated it would be for selected staff only, as an evaluation exercise. We were very sceptical, management were always saying things but never doing them. But evaluation exercise could mean it was not going to cost them a lot. I felt that if it was to happen I might stand a chance, I was by far the youngest on the station and had been an NCO in the army. I dare not let on to anyone, but I was excited, hoping that for once 'Rumour Control' had got it right.

Two weeks later a buff coloured envelope, postmarked County Hall, dropped through my letter box. We assumed it was the rates, but instead it was a letter from the County Medical Officer. In terse terms the aforementioned informed me I had been selected to attend the County Hospital for one week's experimental resuscitation training. They must have held high level financial talks with the Treasurer's Department, for the letter also went on to state that I would receive full pay, less shift allowance. I could also claim second class rail fare, in arrears, on production of used tickets. As a certain doctor had decided my town did not need a rail link many years before, I thought it best to use my car for the eighty mile a day round trip. It seemed common sense to me so I never bothered to ask, I later discovered I would not be paid for those miles as the expense had not been authorised!

In due course at the appointed hour stated, I found my way to the hospital, and at 0900 hours duly reported to the Sister in charge of the Hospital Casualty Department. My first problem of that week began at 0901 hours.

In those days, and I am sure it is still the same today, young nurses were the target for single ambulancemen to chat up. Eventually they all seemed to marry Doctors or ambulancemen. Nurses were always helpful to us in getting a patient through a clinic quickly, or a safe bet for a cup of tea at nights on the ward, and perfect for getting rid of an awkward patient. In fact we all appreciated nurses and thought the world of them. But, unless they went off to have babies and return part time as middle aged mums to earn a few bob and look after ambulancemen with pots of tea, at some point in their careers they would swap a pale blue dress for a navy blue dress and, generally, undergo a personality change. And didn't we know it when they did!

The sight of a stately form in a navy blue uniform, starched white apron over a prominent bosom and the manner of a Regimental Sergeant Major bearing down on me, made me realise I had found the Sister in charge of the Hospital Casualty Department. Or rather, she had found me. Sister was well aware it was she who was "In Charge"! The imposing woman looked down her nose at me with undisguised dislike and asked frostily "May I help you, this is the staff entrance, sir." The Sister had a way of pronouncing the word 'SIR'. I gave one of my disarming smiles, which I knew at once would not work, and stammered who I was. Sister looked at me as though a foul smell was emanating. Steely eyes moved from my head to my feet and back again. She at last spoke and asked where was my uniform. Blushing I replied I had not been issued with one and received a long lecture on how I would confuse her patients. I wondered about that logic later, for I was dressed in a white coat all week! At last, making it very clear she did not agree with ambulancemen cluttering up her department, and forbidding me to talk to any of her nurses, Sister took me through to meet the Casualty

Doctor. She majestically swept through the department with me scurrying behind, clearly determined to show me that it was her department and not the hospital's!

The Casualty Doctor was one of the nicest men I have ever met; a little guy with a shiny bald head peeping through a ring of black hair. His eyes were deceptively mild behind half moon specs, which were always low on a button nose. With his round pink face, which looked as though he had yet to start shaving, together with a habit of sucking his little fingernail, the doctor looked like a small schoolboy. I was quickly to learn this was a false image, carefully cultivated over many years. That doctor was a pioneer in the field of ambulance training. It is a great shame he never lived to see the Service today; it was men like him who brought about the transition from 'snatch-and-run' to paramedic. I learned later that little doctor had fought long and hard to pioneer ambulance training in his department, and, unbeknown to me, I was his first guinea pig. He was most concerned that ambulance crews were on the road without any form of training or medical knowledge, not just for our sake but the sake of the patients. His favourite comment, spoken with a twinkle in his eye, was:

"I'm not bothered about you lot, nor the patients – it's the work for me putting it right afterwards! If I can teach you deadbeats to do it correctly, I can retire!"

I spent the whole day at the Doctor's side, learning from him with every patient. By mid-afternoon he had me examining patients and giving my diagnosis before he gave his. He would pass me an x-ray and, like training a dog, say 'Find it lad!' By the end of the week, I was getting good. Not only was the Doctor my teacher but he protected me from Sister, who, he admitted, frightened him also. He once confided that when he had first moved to the hospital she had been a very pretty staff nurse and he had been tempted to ask her out. Pulling a face he muttered "Look what I missed!"

Tuesday morning saw me in Theatre for the day. Scrubbed, capped and gowned, I watched the insides of people in controlled circumstances – instead of laid by the roadside. Whilst some of the 'old school' surgeons ignored me, the newer ones seemed to delight in showing off their skills. It was fortunate that the Sister in charge of that section was as enthusiastic about my attendance as the casualty doctor; it was she who took time and trouble explaining things to me. Apart from the interest of seeing the Theatre in action, it was invaluable for me to be able to watch the process of airway management of an unconscious patient in a controlled situation. I also had their recovery explained to me and learned more about oxygen, airways and the factors affecting them. The week flew by, and even though it entailed early starts and late finishes, I enjoyed every minute. I learnt a lot and made good friends. The fact that I had made no attempt to attack any nurse within the Casualty Department even evoked what I took to be a faint smile from Sister on the Friday... but a nurse said it was 'just wind'!

On Saturday I was back at work. The number of hours at the hospital did not count towards my working week, and I was due to do a late shift. I was on with Jack, who was now only months away from retirement. Jack was well 'past it' and had no interest left in the job. He had seen it all, and like an old dog he was not impressed with the enthusiasm of a "young 'un". It was a very quiet shift; I read my text book and notes, Jack went to sleep. As always happened, we had just opened our sandwiches and started tea when the emergency telephone rang – a motorbike had hit a car. I was driver, because Jack didn't like to drive. I knew I would also be attendant at the scene for he didn't like to get involved with patients either! It annoyed me intensely at the time, but I realise now that at 64 years of age I would not like to be an operational ambulanceman. With the bell on the bumper ringing, the Bedford bounced down the road as I built up speed to a flat out 70mph. It was fast enough for the roads in those days. It was far too fast for Jack, who was hanging onto the panic bar and grumbling.

We arrived at the scene of the accident and with bursts of the bell I weaved the ambulance past the line of held-up cars to reach the patient. It was the usual confusion, a bike in bits in the middle of the road, a dented car, lots of people standing around with arms folded, waiting for the arrival of us and the police. The car driver was not hurt and immediately started to tell me it was not his fault, and that the bike had been on the wrong side of the road. I responded that I didn't need to know and that he should tell the police, who would soon be there. Leaving him most dissatisfied, I went to the youthful motorcyclist who was sitting on a box by the kerb. The young chap said he was shaken up but not in any pain. Apart from a nasty case of gravel rash down the side of his face where he had made close contact with the road, there seemed to be little wrong with him. I had just started to examine the lad when up came a helpful member of the public with a cup of tea. As he held out his hand to take the cup, my newly-gained knowledge as a trained ambulanceman came to the fore.

"Sorry Madam, he can't have that. The patient may need a general anaesthetic later."

The old lady, who clearly thought she was being most helpful, stood looking bewildered, the tea, in what was obviously one of her best cups and saucers, shaking in her hand.

"Whatever shall I do with this?" she asked. Before I could speak, Jack stepped forward, hand outstretched.

"Give us it 'ere Missus!" With that, and to my great embarrassment, Jack stood amidst the chaos of the RTA and slowly drank the cup of tea!

CHAPTER NINE

The Greatcoat

I recall the words of an old army song, 'Then you're issued with your kit, a uniform that doesn't fit'. I was to discover that this was also very applicable to the Ambulance Service...

I had been in the service for about six months. I had already had a telephone installed at my home so that I could join the 'standby rota'. In the mid-sixties, a telephone was still a bit of a status symbol, and neither my wife nor I had got over the novelty of it. We both leapt up when it rang in the middle of the morning. The old Leading Hand was as grumpy as ever.

"Come an' tek this uniform 'ome, it's gerrin in the way!"

I was on my bike and off like a shot to the station.

Everything was in a large cardboard box. Although the contents were listed and checked by HQ stores, the old fool insisted on opening the sealed box and counting the items before allowing me to sign for the contents. All the time he was, as usual, puffing at a wizened, hand-rolled cigarette which protruded from under his straggly 'tash, and he continually blew ash over my new uniform. In addition to this I was concerned in case 'grot' from his own ill fitting and shabby uniform fell onto mine. Alongside his tunic, with its range of beer and food stains from years of abuse, mine was delightfully pristine, and the thought of contamination worried me! Of course, having been removed and checked, the contents wouldn't fit back into the box properly, and my cycle ride home was a little fraught, with the bulging box balancing precariously on the handlebars.

I felt like a kid at Christmas as I excitedly pulled items out of the box. My young son claimed the cap and ran out happily to play in it whilst the dog attempted to make a nest in the greatcoat. I had to admit to a growing disappointment. I should have known that like all the others it would be a poor fit, the word 'tailoring' being more obvious on the makers label than in the garment's make up. The trousers reached under my arms whilst the tunic sleeves covered my hands. Each chrome button, bearing the County Arms, was sewn at a different angle. They used to talk about 'Friday afternoon cars', well this must have been made late Saturday night in a boozer!

Luckily, my wife was able to do something, as I desperately wanted to wear the uniform, and from the tales I had heard, anything returned for alteration was lost for ever. After a lot of hard sewing and much effort with an iron and damp cloth, the tunic and trousers looked something like a fit. I eventually dressed in the entire uniform for the first time, feeling as pleased as Punch, though, thinking back, it was like most civilian uniforms of the day, thick navy blue serge, silver buttons, blue shirt and black tie, all topped with a peaked cap.

The following morning I went to work looking like an ambulanceman for the first time... well, at least the shoulder epaulette said so!

That uniform transformed my working life; no longer was I chased from hospital departments or mistaken for an insurance man. Of course, it also had its disadvantages. The Service must have bought a lot of cheap shirts, for the garments were all enormous around the body and in the arm. In addition, they all had loose collars. I had never owned a shirt with separate collars before, and having to use front and back studs took a little getting used too. Still, I felt the part, and was most offended when, halfway through my first uniformed shift, I lifted a small girl out of the ambulance and she vomited down the front of my tunic!

I had already been taught all the methods of dealing with the range of stains we encountered daily, within days instructed on the quickest method of removing blood, an occupational hazard. Sadly, it was not long before the newness wore off my pristine uniform. The blood and vomit could be removed, but it never looked the same. What is more, a few RTA's ensured that I was splashed with anti-freeze and had knelt in pools of oil. The uniform quickly developed that 'lived in' look, and no matter how long I spent cleaning and pressing, the cheap material soon looked worn – and it had to last me two years!

However, I was very proud of the greatcoat; this was long before the days of anoraks. We had a navy blue unmarked civilian-style gabardine raincoat, which quickly went shiny, and a greatcoat for winter. They must have slipped up making my overcoat, not only was it an excellent fit but it was made from a lovely smooth material and looked very smart. It was also very warm. Naturally, it was midsummer when it was issued, but when winter came around it proved to be magnificent. The first time I wore it though, I found it could be too warm!

Winter had come early, it was November and bitterly cold. I was on late shift with Ian, we had finished all the jobs for the day and were relaxing in the office listening to the radio. In those days there were no TV sets on stations, so the only form of entertainment, apart from talking or reading, was the radio. We had a slight problem here, because our station did not have one, but one day we discovered that Godly Green had 'acquired' one (where it came from was a mystery, but knowing Godly, he would not have bought it). He would shut himself in his office and listen, with the volume set very low. When he went home at night the set would be locked away in a cupboard. Smithy was the first to find out about it, and word quickly spread. When the L/A went at six, a spare key, which had been 'acquired', was taken from its hiding place and the radio retrieved. The night crew would ensure that it was locked away before they left in the morning and Godly was never any the wiser.

That evening, whilst drinking the inevitable mug of tea and listening to a play, we received a call to attend to a patient who had collapsed. Struggling into greatcoats and caps as we hurried to the 'bus', we were soon mobile and speeding to the scene. As the attendant, I had the full-time job of clearing the inside of the windscreen, as the night was so cold. The heaters emitted warm air in summer but they took a long time to warm up in the winter expecting them to de-mist the windscreen was a forlorn hope.

We arrived at the call, a small terraced house in a narrow street, and were met at the door by an agitated old lady. She had called the doctor but as he had not arrived she had called us. We followed her and found her husband collapsed in front of a roaring fire. Although he was still warm (probably from the fire) the old gentleman looked as though he had died as soon as he hit the carpet. Our job, however, was to save life, so we immediately set to work. Ian fixed the mechanical oxygen machine onto the patient's mouth and nose, I knelt by his side and started cardiac massage. After a few minutes it became obvious that he had 'gone' and we were not going to revive him. It's difficult in a situation like that to stop and break the news to a relative, especially one so old, alone and frightened, when they are clearly hoping against hope that we can perform a miracle. Just as I looked towards Ian for guidance, we heard the door bell and the old lady shuffled away to answer it. We paused and stretched our aching backs, sweat pouring from us. To perform cardiac massage and resuscitation effectively is hard work and it takes it out of you, and it is not made any easier when wearing greatcoats next to a roaring fire.

The old lady ushered in the doctor. We knew him well, a big and burly old Irishman. He knelt by our side and, greeting us, requested we stop whilst he placed his stethoscope on the patient's chest. He listened for a full minute before his eyes caught mine, and with a hardly perceptible movement of his head he confirmed what we already knew. Rising to his feet he spoke.

"Will you be trying for a minute more lads?"

We went back to work whilst the GP started to talk in a gentle way to the old lady. The heat was building, sweat was now running down my back, my shirt sticking, beads of sweat dripping from my nose. Ian's chubby face looked the same. We heard a match strike as the doctor lit his pipe.

"It's a grand job you're doing there lads, oy wish oy could be as clever as you fellas."

Gently, he told the old lady that her husband had gone and asked us to stop, knowing if we continued our efforts much longer he would have had two more collapse cases to deal with.

We transferred the patient into the front room, Ian went next door to fetch a neighbour to look after the old lady whilst the doctor telephoned the undertaker. We were collecting our kit when the doctor stood by my side. His kindly face crinkled into a grin and I could not help but notice that he seemed to have hair growing out of every bit of his face. He reached over and with finger and thumb felt the lapel of my greatcoat.

"Tis a grand bit o' cloth ye have there me owd son. When ye part we it, oid like it for me dog to slape on!"

CHAPTER TEN

It Could Happen to Anyone

He was a disaster magnet. If something was going to go wrong, it would wait for him to come on duty and sign on. He attracted accidents as though they were going out of fashion. He was a very likeable bloke, good company and an interesting talker. He was also a very good ambulanceman, and believed in taking great care of his patients, and me. When you did a shift with Smithy, you could be assured there would be a story to relate.

Everyone had told me about Smithy, he was the standard joke on the station. Smithy freely admitted he was accident prone and said his wife only stayed with him "cause she likes a good laugh." A small man, he was inclined toward being overweight, not fat, just tubby – built for comfort rather than speed.

"Inside this chunky body there's a fat man trying to get out!" was a pearl of wisdom Smithy would often use as he tucked into the enormous meal his wife had provided. We all took sandwiches to work or bought a meat pie but not Smithy, his wife fed him well. He was as bald as could be, but had the most magnificent beard, almost as though his head was on upside down. The beard was always groomed and trimmed to perfection, the sort of whiskers you only saw on a cigarette packet. Smithy always said the navy used to refer to them as a 'full set'. He was very proud of his beard. Someone had said it made him look distinguished, and since that day he had taken great care of it, nurturing and grooming those flowing whiskers. It was a well known fact that people noticed him, and because of the beard, they remembered him, saying that 'it had happened when they were with the bearded guy'.

Having heard so much about Smithy, I was a little unsure of myself when I reported for a late turn and found he was to be my mate for the shift. Noddy scowled at us and seemed disappointed there were no details outstanding.

"Yer aint got nufink ter do," he said, "Gera grip uda bus."

We took it he meant us to clean the ambulance whilst we waited for any emergency to come. As we didn't usually work together, Smithy and I had to use the relief vehicle. This was the oldest on the station and was rather tatty in comparison with the others. None of the vehicles were too bad, but call sign Hotel was on its last legs, almost worn out – it would do the job but little more. Smithy told me that we should look busy and keep out of the way of those in the office.

We had been pottering about inside the ambulance for about half an hour when Noddy crept over with a detail. He seemed disappointed that he had not caught us doing nothing, which was only because whilst we had been sat talking we could watch the office through the dark glass of the interior. The job was a discharge from the General Hospital to a village out of town, a Mr Jones who lived at

20 Main Street, which would not be too hard to find. 'Hotel' coughed, spluttered and eventually struggled into life, and in a cloud black smoke we lurched out of the yard, demonstrating that my driving was not as good as I had thought. However, the ambulance began to behave itself as we proceeded sedately down the road to the hospital. All the time Smithy sang to himself, some wag once said that since he had grown the beard he fancied himself as an opera singer, but Smithy didn't sound like one though! We arrived at the appropriate hospital entrance and entered the ward with our stretcher. On our way to the Sister's office Smithy chatted cheerfully to each patient and nurse we passed; like most ambulancemen he seemed to know everyone.

Sister was not on the ward, but a young nurse pointed to a bed and said that was the patient to go home.

"Mr Jones? Mr Jones of Main Street?" Smithy asked the recumbent patient. The little old man in the bed peered at him short-sightedly.

"You what?" he asked, cupping a hand to an ear. "Have you come to give me a bed bath?"

"No boss, we're going to take you home" said Smithy, "Are you Mr Jones?"

The old man nodded his head.

"Mr Jones, Main Street, 20 Main Street?" Smithy shouted again into his ear. The face screwed up and a shaking hand went to the other ear as it twisted toward us.

"You what?"

Smithy repeated the question. This time we were in luck and the old man nodded frantically. As usual at that time of the evening, all nurses were busy rushing around to get their work finished before the late shift came on duty. I caught one as she rushed past and checked that it was the correct patient, she assured me he was waiting to go home and pointed to his case and a paper bag of dressings. Good enough for us. We loaded Mr Jones onto the stretcher and with waves at everyone we left the ward and proceeded to the ambulance.

Smithy sat in the back and tried to chat to the old man. As the patient was stone deaf he sang to him. (The patient may have enjoyed the song but I was pleased there was a glass bulkhead between us!) Reaching the village in the gathering gloom, I slowed down as I looked for the house. Smithy slid the partition open and told me the patient had said it was a white house set well back from the road. He was right, there it was, a posh carved oak nameplate and under it a number, a number 20 – we'd found his home. I didn't back up the drive, it was not very wide and reverse took a bit of finding on the old lady. I didn't want to show myself up. Gathering the patient's belongings I walked to the front door. It was a most impressive house and as I rang the doorbell I heard the melodious chimes echo through the house. Nobody came, and after a few more tunes on the bell I tried the door and found it open. I shouted a few times but there was no reply, it was clear no one was at home. I returned to the ambulance and together we shouted at the patient. Eventually we got through to him and he understood, he said his daughter would still be at work and we should put him to bed.

We carried the patient into the spacious hall and upstairs, he told us the second room on the left. The bedroom was like those you see in magazines in the dentist's waiting room, all drapes, frilly cushions and expensive furniture.

"Are you sure this is your room pop?" Smithy shouted.

The old man assured him it was, so we put him to bed. I asked if he had his daughter's telephone number so that we could ring her. Asking what time it was the old man said she would be home soon, he'd be alright but would we make him a cup of tea. Smithy sat with the him whilst I found the kitchen. Putting on the kettle, I hunted around the oak units until I found the makings for tea for our patient. I took him up a cup and was pleased when he insisted we join him. We all sat in the posh bedroom whilst drinking tea from expensive china cups and saucers. Afterwards we cleared up and returned everything to the kitchen.

We were both a little concerned about leaving him alone but the old chap insisted his daughter would be home very soon and he would be quite safe. He looked nice and comfy so we bid him goodnight and started our return to station. We were about five miles out of the village when Control called and asked if we had cleared Mr Jones yet. Smithy replied yes, he was tucked up in bed.

A few minutes later they came back and asked were we sure. Damn silly question, of course we were sure, Control often got it wrong though, so Smithy slowly and carefully explained what we had done. There was a long pause. Were we sure? Yes we were. Another pause. The radio crackled into life, "Control to Hotel". Smithy answered. "We seem to have a problem, the patient's daughter said he has not come home. I've checked the ward and they said he has gone, you also said he has. This is confusing, would you return to the address and sort it out?" We both swore, I swung the ambulance around and returned to the village.

I pulled up outside the house, which now showed signs of life and together we crunched up the gravel drive, Smithy banged on the door. It was opened a moment later by a most attractive lady. She was a cracker, every inch the well-brought-up type who would live in a posh place like this, looking as though she was a model and dressed like one. Seeing our uniforms, a look of concern crossed her pretty face. Smithy found his voice first. With one of his better smiles he respectfully touched the peak of his cap.

"Good evening madam, I understand you have a problem." The woman frowned and shook her head, saying nothing.

"I understand you've lost your dad?" Smithy continued.

The frown deepened.

"Well", she replied, "I lost him about five years ago. My mother is still alive in London though."

Smithy put on his 'speaking to thickos and noisy kids' type of voice.

"But madam, I can assure you he's in bed, no doubt wanting his tea by now."

Her expression changed from one of concern to one of 'stop messing me about'.

"Who are you my man, and whatever are you doing at my door talking such rubbish? Let me tell you I am a friend of your Chief Constable."

It was not unusual for us to be mistaken for coppers in our navy uniform and silver buttons, but this lady sounded as though she was a bit of a nutcase, not fair for her to be in charge of a nice old guy like her dad. I moved closer to Smithy to support him.

"Madam, we are not officers of the law, so please don't try to bully us. My colleague is telling the truth, we've just returned your dad and put him to bed."

She looked from one to the other of us, beginning to look frightened. At last she spoke.

"If you don't go away, I'll call the police."

Smithy decided at this point that he should try to pacify her and explained, "Madam we're an ambulance crew, we have just returned your dad from the hospital. As you were out we put him to bed. He did say you would be home very soon". The woman looked at each of us unsure of what to do or say. Smithy took the opportunity to speak again.

"May I suggest we clear this up by taking you up to your dad, if we go up to his room you will see him. Come along". With that Smithy pushed past her and went up the stairs. Astonished, she followed, I brought up the rear. Smithy threw open the bedroom door with a flourish, the woman cautiously peeped around and saw her dad fast asleep, but she did not welcome him, in fact her words were.

"Who the hell is *he*?"

I began to get the feeling things were not going according to plan!

It was all very simple really, but it did take some time on the telephone to sort things out. Everyone was most confused, the only one who did not seem to care was the old man. It materialised that on the ward there were two Mr Jones, and both, by the strangest of coincidences lived at 20 Main Street, but in different villages. Our Mr Jones was confused, and the other Mr Jones had not worried that nobody had come for him and had said nothing. The Sister in charge had been off the ward and so the mistake went unnoticed. Our Mr Jones's daughter had checked with the hospital and had worried when they told that her dad had gone. Our posh lady had come home, unaware a strange man was in her bed. Needless to say she was confused when two silly men in uniform had knocked at the door and started to talk a lot of rubbish about her long deceased dad.

At long last everything was sorted out and we took the patient out of bed and to his correct address. It could only have happened to Smithy!

CHAPTER ELEVEN

The Docks

The wind carried sleet and freezing snow from the depth of the North Sea, whipping our coat tails and trying to blow our caps into the river. It was a damn silly place to be on a winter's night.

It had just turned six, Smithy and I thought we'd finished for the day. The cold November day had never really seen daylight, snow was in the air, we had been expecting it all day. When we had to get out of the ambulance, and that was often, for we were on outpatient duties, we were pleased to have our voluminous greatcoats. We had dropped off our last patient and were only a mile from the station.

We had both 'had enough' and were silent, thinking of home and tea, when Control called. Would we return to the General and work a discharge? Of course, they added the usual touch of blackmail.

"He's been waiting a long time, and if you can't do it he'll have a lot longer wait."

We gave a joint sigh and I started to take the details as Smithy swung the Bedford around and pointed the bonnet away from home as we made our way back to the hospital.

By the time we arrived at the General there was no one left in the large outpatients hall, apart from a porter reading a paper, a cleaner trying to make it look something like respectable for the next day, and our patient. We looked twice at him, he was a massive chunk of a man. I suppose the chap had the sort of blond good looks that attract women. A good six feet tall, and as broad as he was long, there was not an ounce of fat on him, clearly all muscle. His lower leg was encased in a plaster cast. We walked over and Smithy said "How do".

The man grunted something we couldn't understand but with patient questioning we slowly discovered he was a Scandinavian seaman and his ship was at the docks about ten mile along the coast. His English was poor but he made himself understood, by saying in a loud booming voice, "Ome, I go ome."

We wheeled him out the department into the back of the ambulance. We opened the rear doors and, before we could attempt to lift him, the giant pushed himself onto his good foot and indicated we move closer. Then, an arm like a tree trunk thumped around our necks and with a push, that had our knees buckling, he swung into the vehicle.

As the attendant, I sat in the back and we attempted to have a form of conversation. The patient in broken English, me in what I thought might sound like Scandinavian. He was looking forward to returning to his ship, which was due to sail that night, he indicated he would be able to do his job with a pot leg. The thought of him at sea working with a plastered leg sounded pretty hairy to me and I tried to explain he should rest, but it was of no use he either did not understand or didn't want to. We had been on the dock a few times before to collect people, but had always had directions. As a result we had little idea of where ships could be found, naturally the patient had none. It's always the same when you are trying to find something in the dark – everywhere is deserted and the only other people you meet are foreign or lost themselves. At last, more by luck than judgement, we found the ship. It was berthed at the end of a long jetty and looked little more than an illuminated toy it was so far away. Our man indicated he would walk, but we insisted that we take him on the carry chair. An ambulance carrychair is a clever item of kit, folds flat for storage but when opened it can be used to move patients in all kinds of situations. Two small wheels allowed it to be tipped back and pushed on the flat. They were ideal for ambulance crew, but not built for patient comfort.

When we got the man on the chair it vanished under his bulk. Smithy, tipped the chair back and with a struggle started to push, whilst he did so I supported the pot leg. The jetty was primarily a means of taking a large pipe out to a ship at the end. Alongside this pipe ran a narrow plank walkway, a low fence along one side, the pipe the other. It did not look safe to our non-seaman's eyes. The planks ran across the jetty with a gap between and we found the tiny wheels of the chair bumped over the gaps. Each bump must have caused the patient's leg to jar but the big man said nothing for the whole of the journey.

It had been cold all day on shore but we quickly found, as we trundled out over that stretch of sea, that the further we went the more the wind came into it's own. It was bitterly cold and we leaned into the wind which attempted not only to take our caps away but blow us off the jetty. We gamely struggled on. Bump, bump, bump went the chair bouncing the poor man along. We could feel every bump as much as he but the guy made no complaint. Every few yards he would shout above the wind "Bloory cold Yar?" We agreed but not in such printable terms. The journey along that exposed jetty seemed endless. Looking down through the planks we could see black icy waters swirling far below us, the wind still trying its hardest to blow us off and into that water. As the fencing was only knee high we were not at all happy with the situation. Smithy was an enthusiastic fair weather sailor with the boat club on the local reservoir but this was not his cup of tea at all. As for me, I was scared stiff!

We seemed to have walked miles and still the ship looked far away, but at last we looked up and saw that the jetty had expanded into a platform; we'd made it. The ship loomed high above us. High! It was like a block of flats with no windows, just wet black steel stretching up as far as we could see. Apart from one light on the platform it was dark, as black as pitch. We could see the top of the ship for it was well illuminated, but that wasn't a lot of use to us down there. We looked around in dismay and I said something silly like "Where's the door?" or "Shouldn't there be some steps?"

With that, and to our horror, our patient pointed to a rope ladder dangling and swaying against the ship's side, it was made of thick rope with wooden steps, each about two feet apart.

"Bloory oop thar" he announced, pointing to the swaying ladder. Smithy and I looked at the ladder in horror, then we looked at him. The guy must have been at least eighteen stone not counting the weight of that pot leg. We could never manage to carry anyone up that ladder, not even on a good day, never mind in this weather.

"Sorry me old mate" Smithy said, scratching the side of his nose, "We'll have to take you back to the hospital until they can arrange for help from the dock or the Fire Service, or something."

For a moment I thought the man was going to explode with fury. Then he reached up, grabbing the front of my greatcoat, for a second I thought he was going to push me into the water. With a heave that almost had me on top of him he pulled himself up.

"Blurry go oop, blurry go ome!"

With that our patient grabbed hold of the rope ladder. Using both hands and his one good leg, the pot swinging he started to climb. We looked on in trepidation and fear. His weight and the gusting wind made the ladder sway alarmingly. We thought that any moment he would fall. Thoughts rushed through my mind. He would kill himself if he fell. That would give us no end of problems as he was still in our care. Worse still if he fell he might land on us on the small jetty. That would be a disaster! Perhaps if he fell into the water between the ship and jetty it would soften his fall, but with that pot on his leg he would go straight to the bottom! My thoughts were summed up as Smithy spoke.

"The prat's gonna kill himself! He'll never get up there!"

At that point, the seaman stopped and we both felt panic rise. He hung there, swaying in the wind as it tried to carry him away. The pot leg held out from the side of the ship.

"Hell he's going to fall off the darn thing!" Smithy breathed.

The man looked down at us, face in shadow. He shouted but the wind carried his voice away. Again he shouted. Did he want help? What could we do in the situation? The giant took one faltering step down a rung and shouted again, again we could not hear. What on earth were we to do! At that point the wind dropped for a moment, he grabbed the opportunity and called out again. This time we caught his words.

"Coom oop men. I give you blurry beer!"

We politely declined...

CHAPTER TWELVE

Change

The Service thrived on rumour. I'm sure some were started because there were no rumours around at the time. The fact the Service covered a large county with scattered stations was partly to do with it, for staff never met each other. The other factor was that ambulancemen thrive on gossip. Encouraged by long periods of inactivity at stations and hospitals, you had to talk about something.

I had been in the service almost a year, a year in which time I'd changed from a naive and rather shy young man to one who now knew he had to take command of situations and attempt to gain order from chaos. I had grown up quickly and had learned a lot about people: how they interact, how they behave under stress when pushed into unexpected situations, or when in distress. I had gained a lot in knowledge and confidence, the job had seen to that.

It was a rare event to go outside our own patch, but on the very odd occasion a run would come up that took us to places and meet men from other stations. When we did, it was amazing what you learned. One thing I learned which rankled was that I seemed to be at one of the worst stations. At some places, it appeared, management actually helped the ambulance crews to work! Occasionally we would get to Ambulance Headquarters. Now that *was* the place for gossip! The HQ lads thought themselves the tops, and I'm sure they invented most of the rumours to keep up this image. We hardly ever met them and knew Controllers only by their voices over the radio. I never gave HQ a great deal of thought, and didn't know what I expected it to be like. I had a vague feeling that HQ must be very smart and impressive. I never expected it to be a bit like the place I found on my first visit. It came as a shock. County Ambulance HQ was a rather grandiose name for a redundant block of ex-military buildings. It must have been a transport unit, for it consisted, in the main, of a long row of garages with a single block of office and domestic accommodation. Everything was rather tatty and disappointing, not a bit as I had imagined.

I had been to the nearby hospital and whilst waiting for my patients had been ordered to HQ to collect stores for our station. I followed their directions and had it not been for the faded sign and parked ambulances, I would have missed the place. I looked around in amazement as I parked in the yard and found my way to the control room. Again, a shock. I don't know what I had expected but certainly something better than what I actually found.

It was a warm day, and the door was propped open with a telephone directory, I knocked and entered. The shabby room was furnished with old chairs and tables, nothing matched. Every surface was piled high with books and assorted paperwork, most looking as though it had been undisturbed for years. One wall was covered with a large and faded map of the county, each town identified by a worn out section where countless fingers had rubbed over that part to identify somewhere; every other inch of wall space was taken by notices and posters of varying degrees of age and shades of yellow. The floor was covered by an old carpet which must have graced a posh house many years before, but was now threadbare and tattered. Under all tables and chairs the dust was piled high. In the centre of the room was a large table, again covered in junk. In the middle of this table was a radio controller and microphone, looking little different to the unit at our station. The rest of the table was taken up by an obviously home made wooden shelving system, slots containing booking and detail sheets. The image was not helped by a pile of books supporting one side of the fixture, a cupboard unit from an old ambulance holding up the other. The rest of the desk was taken by well thumbed exercise books and telephones. I had never seen so many phones in one place before. There must have been seven or eight telephone handsets on that desk, it was clearly apparent that each had been added as the need arose for an additional line. All were of differing shapes and colours, from shiny new to old black, new ivory to aged yellow (in those days you only had the choice of a black or white telephone). The wires of these were twisted together across the desk like mating snakes. In one corner of the table they met and went up to the ceiling bound together with string and sticky tape, looking like a knotted umbilical cord. These then looped across the yellow, smoke-stained ceiling, supported by a range of nails, cup hooks and sticking plasters. Eventually this accumulation reached the wall and disappeared through a roughly hewn hole. A polite description for the whole place was 'tatty'. A large hunch-backed man in shirtsleeves, two chrome bars on each shoulder, looked up and smiled. As soon as he spoke I recognised the voice as Jacko, one of the nicer guys. Jacko immediately made me very welcome, swinging his arm to illustrate the place and apologised for the room's condition, it was obviously an embarrassment to him. It looked to be a horrible place to have to work. His next words took me aback.

"Of course it's bound to improve when we get the new boss. Can't make it any worse can he?"

This was red hot news and my ears pricked up. I had heard that if you wanted anything spread around the Service all you had to do was to tell Jacko and say keep it a secret. He obviously took great delight telling me that the CAO had decided to retire only that day and a new man would soon be in post. He then went on to discuss the faults of all the other officers in the Service, it was rewarding to learn that HQ didn't have a good opinion of Godly Green. Jacko was adamant the post had to go to an outsider. I could not wait to get back to my station to spread the news! Jacko sent me to the crew room where I met the two men on duty. Over a cuppa, they hinted the Deputy had no chance of taking over as he had upset too many people at County Hall, it was also hinted, with knowing looks, that he was 'looking after too many women.' They too were looking forward to change. I thought about the elderly silent old man I had met just once at interview, and his cup of tea I had drunk. The Chief had not impressed me, and I was sure the Service must improve with a change of boss. At this point Jacko telephoned to say my patients were ready, so I bade farewell, collected the supplies from a very helpful old lady in 'Admin' – which was in a similar condition to 'Control' – and departed.

I walked into the station office on my return and took great delight in mentioning the news regarding the CAO to Noddy. The watery eyes bulged behind his dirty glasses and fag ash was coughed in my direction.

"Ah yer shore?" he demanded.

Giving the impression I had a number of secrets tucked away, I nodded.

"Go git yer bus filled wi juice" was all he said.

Before I was out of the door Noddy was racing into Godly's office, shouting "Mr Green, Mr Green, have you heard the news?"

I hoped it spoilt their tea!

The news spread like wildfire, and next day, when I reported on duty, everyone wanted more details. It was soon very noticeable that Godly Green believed he would get the job, for he started to throw his weight about. The two Leading Hands, who were both scared stiff of Godly when all was well, could not take the excitement and started to panic. In the matter of a few days they were both a bundle of nerves. Even in those lax days it seemed incredible that anyone would appoint Godly to the job. Whilst we had no idea what the post of Chief Ambulance Officer entailed, we were well aware Godly was not capable of the undertaking. The man had demonstrated that it was only because we got on with the job, despite his blundering that he was able to run even the one station. The situation regarding Godly's promotion chances was not helped by Ted encouraging him to develop greater aspirations of promotion and grandeur.

Since starting in the service, Ted had managed to become Godly's favourite. Everyone on the station, apart from the three in the office, knew Ted was 'taking the Mickey', but nevertheless he had a knack of getting into Godly's good books. Although a born comedian, Ted had a long mournful face, and years as an undertaker had enabled him to adopt an immediate look of concern and compassion. This worked well when dealing with patients, and it also worked in his favour when he 'wound up the three deadbeats'. The fact Ted had been in the Brigade of Guards, and a sergeant at that, ensured Godly thought him to be someone special. When Ted hinted to Green that he had a medal, Godly almost fawned over him. Ted told the rest of us that he had four medals, but all for campaigns rather than valour. But if Mr Green chose to misunderstand and think a member of his staff was something special then it was not Ted's fault!

Ted quickly convinced Godly that he was the ideal choice for the job of Chief.

"You have the bearing Mr Green, you look the part. When I first saw you I knew you were a born leader of men. In fact at first glance I mistook you for a General I met in the desert, he was your double..."

It seems hard to believe that anyone could give credence to Ted's words but Green beamed and took it all in. How Ted kept a straight face I will never know, but he was enjoying every moment of winding up Godly. But he didn't stop there. Ted also intimated that Noddy should take over Godly's job. The old L/A's face was a picture as Ted buttered him up. We watched this pantomime from afar and enjoyed every moment. The two strutted about like new converts into religion, throwing their weight about to the delight of all. When Ted happened to let it slip that a friend of his was a member of the Health Committee our delight and enjoyment knew no bounds! As the weeks passed it all became too much for poor old Flapper Furguson. The twitch in his left eye became permanent and he would leap when someone shouted or the telephone rang. Finally, Flapper went off sick, with only months to go until his retirement and we never saw him again.

We, of course, heard nothing about what was happening regarding the process of filling the vacancy. We assumed Green had not got the job when Smithy reported one morning that Godly had pulled up outside the office with a squeal of brakes. Instead of his usual routine, he had got out, slammed the car door and stamped into the office, slamming the door. Shouting to Noddy to stuff his effing tea, Godly retreated into his office and slammed that door. The discovery he was acting like a bear with a sore head had us correctly assuming he had not been called for interview. In due course, we learned that the appointment of Chief Ambulance Officer had gone to the Chief of a smaller Service from another county. We considered this to be rather academic and of no interest to us...

How wrong we were!

CHAPTER THIRTEEN

More Changes

"Nice looking place you've got here boy-o, do you enjoy the job?"

The lilting Welsh voice brought me back to reality from my daydream. I made the standard reply.

"Yes it's a good job... would be even better if we didn't have any patients!"

I looked down from my lofty perch. It was a Saturday afternoon, Ian was in Godly's office listening to the football results on the radio. I'd decided to remove the flies, bugs and moths that had committed *hara-kiri* and spoilt the looks of the vehicle front. The ladder was perched precariously against the side of the J1 Bedford whilst I reached around the sign and bell, rubbing hard with a petrol-soaked cloth, removing the grot collected during the week. Whilst the station was tucked well off the side street, hidden from the public, we often had locals dropping in for a chat, we even got the very occasional one who would bring us a home-baked cake. Looking down, I studied the stranger. He was a queer looking guy who I'd never seen before – I would have remembered him for sure. He was very tall and thin as a rail. A thick tweed sports coat hung from his sparse frame like an outsize tent, his thin arms protruding well below his cuffs, ending in enormous hands. His baggy and creased trousers were too short, emphasising his enormous feet that looked like two black barges pointing in almost opposite directions. His face, behind an enormous pair of horn-rimmed spectacles, was thin, with an unhealthy pallor. Apart from a bobbing Adam's apple it was his eyes you noticed; piercing eyes. They shone through his glasses, seeming to look right into you.

"Thought I'd pop in and say 'ello boy-o, have you got the kettle on?"

I looked down at him again. Cheeky sod, I mean we were noted for being a soft touch to most folk, but there was a limit. The man's scrawny neck stuck out of a shirt collar which was miles too big for him, or maybe it was someone else's shirt, it certainly looked as though it had been bought for someone far fatter than him. The stranger had a silly beam on his face, a sort of lopsided grin, and all the time his eyes seemed to bore into me. Then it struck me. I suddenly wondered if he could be a mental patient who had escaped! The way the clothes hung, they all seemed, apart from his trousers, to have been made for a larger man. I felt a touch of unease creeping over me. I decided I'd better chat in case he was about to attack. I felt it would be a lot safer if Ian was with me. Sliding down the ladder, making sure I did not scratch the bus, I smiled at the weird stranger.

"Yeh, good idea, come on in squire."

I kept a careful eye on him as he followed me around the vehicle. The man seemed to be taking a great interest in Sugar, rubbing the paint his fingers. Reaching the County coat of arms, he paused and studied it.

"Do you know what the motto on the badge means bach?"

Naturally I had no idea, my job was to drive the thing, clean it and look after our patients, not look at it.

"I'm told it means 'Up you Jack', but I could be wrong," I quipped.

The stranger looked hard at me but said nothing. As we reached the back of the bus he stopped to look into the interior. I again felt cautious; was he about to attempt to pinch something?

"Have you ever been in one of these things before squire?" I asked, trying to see if he was a regular patient.

"Oh yes, boy-o, I yave that. I've spent many an 'appy hour in one of these things, more time than you I suppose."

Again that lopsided grin, the eyes staring deeply into mine. I felt nervous as he continued to stare hard at me making no effort to speak or move. I stared back, knowing I had to hold my ground. That same inane lopsided grin appeared again followed by a loud piercing chuckle. Then he spoke.

"Don't you know who I yam boy-o?'"

That settled it, he must be a mental case.

"No idea squire, but I'm not a proud fella, I'll talk to anyone. Come and have a cup of tea."

The man didn't move, just stared at me, and a greater feeling of unease crept over me. Should I humour him, should I grab him, should I run? Before I could reach a decision he spoke.

"I thought the grapevine would have warned you kiddo. I yam your new gaffa, I yam the new CAO."

I looked at him in horror.

"Oh my gawd and I've been calling you squire!"

The man's face crumpled into the grin again, he stuck out a huge hand.

"At least you didn't tell me to naff off!"

He followed me into the office and I introduced him to Ian, who looked uncomfortable being caught with the radio. The CAO seemed to be a little surprised to hear it was normally locked away. We gave him a guided tour of the station, during which he said little but clearly missed nothing. After showing him around, we made tea and sat and chatted for some time. An hour later he left with a cheery goodbye. We decided he was a good guy and the Service had to improve under him, agreeing it could not get much worse.

It was only much later we realised that apart from learning he came from a small town in Wales, with an unpronounceable name, and had been Chief of a Welsh Service with an equally tongue twisting name, we knew absolutely nothing about him at all. The worry was, how much had we told him?

Of course, by Monday when we returned to work word had got around and everyone wanted to know what the new Chief was like. We both pretended we knew a great deal, not letting on that we knew next to nothing. We basked in our new glory for some weeks. We knew that Godly Green was dying to ask us about the Chief, but pride would not allow him to speak to such lowly mortals as us. For some months nothing happened, all remained the same as before. The only change was that the radio appeared in the crew room. Noddy told us that Mr Green had thought we should have the loan of it, he couldn't understand why, especially since Noddy's workload had increased since Flapper had not been replaced.

We assumed that any idea of big changes taking place was all talk and nothing concrete was going to happen. Then Godly started going to HQ with great regularity. Naturally, he never told us anything, but would always be in a foul temper on his return. He would spend long periods in his office and longer periods talking on the telephone to the other Station Officers. We suspected something was really happening when Noddy disappeared. He just went. One day he was his usual horrible self, working hard to be as objectionable as possible, upsetting as many people as he could, effing, blinding, blowing fag smoke at all, slurping tea and noisily shouting at anyone who might take notice.

The following morning Noddy was finished, retired, gone without a 'goodbye' or even a burst of foul language! A large canvas sack containing his uniform stood by his locker. Godly told Bill to record it and put it in the store, Bill said he was not touching it, as he might catch something unknown to man and he had not had a jab against Bubonic plague! He chucked it into the heating boiler. We never told Godly.

We never saw Noddy again, he was gone for good and no one would miss him.

The following day the shift crew were amazed to find Godly in the office when they came on duty at eight, sorting the morning runs, or attempting to. Of course, he had no idea what to do, so we all took over and did it ourselves. It was suggested we should leave it to him and let him 'get it in the neck' from Control, but that would have affected the patients and we did not want them to suffer. After that, Godly retreated into his office with the paperwork and went very silent. We almost, but not quite, started to feel sorry for him…

Then it happened, the unthinkable, Godly Green left! One morning 'Taff' as the CAO had come to be known, came to the station with a young Sub-Officer from a station in the north of the county. They went into the inner sanctum with Godly and shut the door. Nothing could be heard, only the sound of voices speaking, sometimes loudly. An hour later Mr Green left the office without a word, but with a look of hate on his bright red face. Clasped to his chest was his briefcase and a cardboard box.

The CAO entered the crew room and introduced the Sub as Alan Barker, who was to take over the station. Having demanded tea for the two of them he said, almost in passing.

"Mr Green has gorn like. 'e come over all funny, 'ad a lot of personal problems of late, like, so I gave 'im the opportunity to go for 'ealth reasons. He's gonna take life a lot easier, 'es been over doin' it of late, like. You lads gonna 'av a whip round for 'im?"

The duty crew looked at the Chief in amazement. With a lopsided grin and the comment of, "Now look after this new boy-o and don't lead him astray like the last one, look you," he left.

Just like that!

The new man, and the CAO, proved to be the best thing that had ever happened to that station and the Service. At long last we felt that someone was beginning to think and to care. Rumours were rife and we learnt that almost all the old guard, who had enjoyed an easy life, had suddenly gone, taken early retirement or left on health grounds. We were all given new responsibilities on the station and Alan, the Sub, started to prove himself. He changed everything, even things that we enjoyed came up for review. We won the odd point, but it had now stopped being a 'them and us' 'win or lose' situation. We enjoyed the new system and worked to make the changes successful.

One major change was that they never replaced the retired Leading Hands. A lot of stuff was sent to HQ and lots of forms, beloved by the old guard, were scrapped. Control became more involved, all calls going directly to them instead of our station. One day a workman turned up and installed a large bell to the outside wall and inside the crew room. Control activated the call out system and when the bell sounded we knew it! You had to become mobile in a hurry to get away from the noise! Rather than wait for telephone connections, we called Control by radio to receive emergency details. This change certainly speeded up turn-out times. That was not the only change to enable us to reach the patient faster, we also got klaxon horns instead of bells. Now cars and trucks heard us coming and could move out of our way. The bells might have sounded better, but they were only of use to cyclists and walkers. The job was suddenly changing out of all recognition. Even the older hands agreed it was a vast improvement. We all started to enjoy life a lot more and everybody mucked in. The best factor was the removal of unpleasant L/As, the next best was the introduction of permanent mates.

I was lucky, I was paired up with a man who had transferred from another station. Pete was an ex-sailor about my own age with a similar amount of service. Pete became my mate in every sense of the word. We not only worked well together, we also became good friends. Pete and I worked as a team, very quickly learning from each other, the most important factor being no matter who was driver or attendant, we each knew what the other was doing. It was the start of a happy working relationship. At last I felt the Service was achieving something for the benefit of patients and the job suddenly became a lot better.

CHAPTER FOURTEEN

The Explosion

The raucous clanging of the emergency bell had us moving immediately. Pete leapt into the cab, started the engine and called Control on the radio whilst I opened the garage doors. As I slammed the doors shut behind the bus and leapt in beside him, Pete let in the clutch and accelerated from the station.

Pete's brow was furrowed as he spoke. "Dunno if Control's having us on, but he said it's an explosion at that posh men's shop at the junction of High Street and Victoria Street. He said a fire crew was on the way."

I looked at Pete in amazement as my foot stamped on the switch for the horns and kept it there. With beacons (we were then very modern) and headlights blazing, the horns heralding our approach, the Bedford J1 thundered down the road. Explosions where unheard of in Britain in those days.

The shop was only a short distance away and we were determined to get there before the Fire Brigade. It was a mid-week morning and the normally busy High Street had little traffic to slow us down. As we swung into Victoria Street we saw the shop and also an excited young man, jumping up and down waving his arms, flagging us down. One look at his wide eyed stare and pale face showed he was in an obvious state of shock and panic. The way he looked, he could quite easily be the next patient for us. As we climbed out of the cab the young man chattered and shouted something incomprehensible as he ran in front of us into the shop. Suddenly, we realised he was shouting over and over again that the Manager had been blown up.

We followed him in to the genteel surroundings of the shop. Everything looked normal, or as normal I assumed it should look – I could hardly afford to look in the window, let alone buy anything from a shop like this. With us following close behind, the young man rushed through the shop and into a room beyond. The immaculate appearance of the shop changed as we walked through a curtain and entered the back room. Piles of cardboard hat boxes and racks of clothes were everywhere, covering every available surface. By the time we passed through another door and reached the foot of the stairs, we had collected another two men and a very young female, all in stages and degrees of shock and hysterics. The girl threw her arms around Pete and burst into tears. Whilst he tried to disentangle himself and calm her, I picked my way around the obstacle course of boxes on the stairs, my professional eye working out the return journey with a patient through the clutter, and deciding what had to be moved. I could hear everyone following me. By now our party had grown to a small and very excited crowd. One of the staff pointed to a door and whispered "In there."

Nobody offered to accompany us through the door. Pete had at last managed to detach himself from the girl, and together we forced open the door and entered the room. We looked around the mess and saw our patient, or rather a part of him. It took a moment to find him for he was under a pile of collapsed wood and plaster. This had obviously been the main bathroom in the days when the property had been one of a street of smart Victorian houses. At some time, probably when the house had been converted into a shop, the large bathroom had been converted into a smaller bathroom, toilet and storeroom, this had been achieved by erecting a wooden frame and covering it with thin plywood and plaster.

The explosion had caused the structure to collapse and the room was back to its original large size. Boxes, clothes, hats and packets of shirts were all over, mixed with large and small bits of wood, all covered with plaster and dust. We could just make out part of the man's legs sticking from below the wreckage. We were delighted at that point to hear the sound of heavy boots indicating the Fire Brigade had arrived. Friendly rivalry is alright, but at a time like this we needed those lads by our side. Together, we lifted the debris off the patient so that Pete and I could attend to him. He was a man of about fifty, unconscious but breathing. Apart from a range of cuts, bruises and a possible fractured upper arm, he had severe burns to his buttocks and the back of his thighs. We were more than a little surprised to find his trousers and underpants down around his ankles. Pete and I cast a puzzled glance at each other. Why had someone removed his pants but not treated his injuries? It was plain the panicking staff were in no state to have done anything, and no one else was around. We dressed the patient's wounds, stabilised his arm, and with the help of the fire crew got him down the stairs and into the ambulance. By then a large crowd had gathered, attracted by the fire appliance, ambulance and the police, who had now arrived. I knew one of the coppers and gave him a quick resume of our patient's injuries before we left for the hospital.

As I looked after our patient, Pete called Control and requested they inform Casualty. Although only a short journey the system worked well, as usual, and when we arrived A&E staff were waiting and the patient was wheeled directly into theatre. Just as we were explaining the nature of the incident and injuries to the surprised Casualty Sister, a receptionist waved a telephone hand set in our direction. We were needed at a road accident well out of town. We hastily loaded our stretcher and leapt into the vehicle, Pete hit the accelerator, I the horn push and we were off again. For the rest of that day we covered one job after another without a break. By chance it just happened that we didn't take anyone else into the Casualty Department for the whole of the shift, so we didn't find out any more details about our patient from the explosion.

Rest days and shift patterns split Pete and I for the rest of the week and it was the following Sunday when we began a late shift again. We were interested in the explosion case, but as so often the incident, no one knew what had happened. That had been one of the few advantages of having Noddy on the station, he could always be relied upon to find out the full details of any gossip. The only information we heard was that the patient had been transferred to a specialist burns unit out of County, so we couldn't find him to satisfy our curiosity. It was the middle of the following week before we learned the story. We met up with the police constable who had been at the incident and he delighted in telling us the full details. It would seem that it was the shop manager's habit to go and have a quiet read of his paper each morning at about ten o'clock. If you think about it of course, the most natural place for any man to read at that time of the day is in the loo. So, on that fateful morning, the manager had picked up his daily and gone off as usual. I felt that perhaps the expression 'gone off' was a rather apt description in the circumstances!

The remainder of the tale is pure conjecture because, despite many enquiries, the full facts never emerged. Well, it's not the sort of thing you brag about is it? The manager, apparently, made himself comfortable and opening his paper took out his cigarettes and lit one. What happened next would also seem to be a natural thing for any man to do under the circumstances. He lifted one cheek of his bottom and dropped the lighted match into the toilet pan. The subsequent investigation by the police disclosed that the cleaner at the shop was a most conscientious lady. It was well known that she had a 'thing' about clean loos. It was almost a fixation to her, it would seem she was always trying out new cleaners, bleaches, germ killers and things that got right around the bends. It was further surmised that the gasses given off by this cocktail, perhaps mixed with natural methane, had produced a flammable gas, which was confined within the toilet pan. Normally this would have dissipated into the atmosphere unnoticed, but on this occasion the gas had built up beneath the toilet lid. As soon as the unfortunate shop manager had raised the lid, and sat down, his bottom had formed a further seal.

It was at this most inopportune time, with the build up of gasses below him, that the unfortunate smoker had chosen to enjoy his morning cigarette. We did hear he made a full recovery and returned to work, but we never learned if it stopped him smoking!

CHAPTER FIFTEEN

Working Together

'Policeman delivers baby' – 'Ambulanceman rescues trapped child' – 'Fireman swims to help'. You have all seen this type of headline. The media love it, it sells papers, and it's true. What the public don't realise is that it happens all of the time. You don't read about it very often because usually, no one tells the press.

I once read somewhere, that during a war, the life of a soldier is 99% boredom and 1% fear. I feel that something similar could be applied to all the Emergency Services. The percentages will be different of course, but I would suggest that percentages of panic, fear and humour, could also be included, in addition to which would be a small proportion to include doing something brave, usually because you didn't think of the risks at the time. An emergency or a major incident to one Emergency Service need not necessarily be so to another. A major fire will require an ambulance to stand-by to protect fire crews, but otherwise will cause little disruption to their daily workload. Civil disorder will be a major task for the police but will only call for the others to be put on alert. An evacuation of a hospital will warrant everyone and will require bus companies as well as ambulances. The list is endless. The Emergency Services in this country always work well together when required. I found that in the main they had little contact during the normal working day but when the 'chips were down' or perhaps 'when the bells went down' and the emergency happened they all turned up and got on with their job, working closely with each other.

I have been involved in two major incidents, both were most harrowing experiences. The volume of people injured, coupled with the initial lack of resources is one of great frustration and anguish. You accept that it takes time to move the required resources to the scene, but when you're there trying to cope, the feeling is one of great hopelessness. It's of no comfort to know that every effort is being made to ensure help is on the way if you are unable to look after everyone. However, every part of the country has a major incident plan, and readers should be assured that as it swings into action everything fits into place. I cannot describe the two incidents I was involved with as they may be recognised and cause distress to people who lost loved ones, so I'll move on to other events.

The Road Traffic Accident (RTA) is where the Services generally meet. Whilst the Police attend all, we only go if there are injuries. In the event of anyone being trapped, the Fire Service are called, being the experts at rescue. A number of incidents stick in my mind involving fire crews; here is one.

The rain was coming down in sheets like the stuff you see in films, so heavy it didn't look real. The screen wipers were fighting a losing battle. It was the end of a long day, we had been working non-stop for the full shift and now we had finished the run. Pete was driving and I was the attendant. We were on the way back to the station, hoping against hope we would not get another job, we'd both had enough for one day. My major task was wiping the mist off the inside of the screen. Heaters and demisters were somewhat of a luxury in those days – the Council spent their cash on more important things like no waiting signs and fancy dustbin wagons. My cap and a bit of rag was in constant use fighting a losing battle with the misted screen. The radio crackled, we groaned as we glanced at each other, we heard Control give our call sign and the word 'Priority'. I reached for the handset. We had another job.

Control requested our position, and as soon as I gave it he passed us the detail: an RTA. A car had left the road and gone down a rail embankment, the Fire Service were on their way. We both groaned, as Pete put his foot down, I switched on the beacon and horns. We knew the location well, it was a narrow road winding between trees, in one place curving sharply as it crossed a bridge over the railway. We guessed he had gone in there, the road would be treacherous with wet leaves at this time of the year. It was also at the farthest edge of our patch, a long run, and this was not the sort of weather to be belting along wet and winding country lanes in an ambulance. Pete made good time, but it must have been fifteen minutes before I called in reporting 'on scene'.

I grabbed my first aid box, pushed my cap firmly down and leapt out of the cab... straight into a deep puddle, both shoes filled with water! Not a good start.

I looked down over the smashed fencing and saw to my horror the car was on its side across the railway tracks.

I pulled open the cab door and before Pete could jump out and shouted to him to tell Control to stop any trains. You will have heard the term. 'I proceeded to the scene'. What it meant, in this instance, was me plunging into waist high, dense, wet undergrowth as I started down the slope. Within two paces, both feet went in opposite directions, I half fell, half stumbled and then ran down the thirty odd feet to the railway track, colliding with every tree on my way down. I reached the tracks out of breath with a twisted ankle, no cap and very, very wet. Hobbling to the car, I saw that it had rolled a number of times, flattening the roof to the waistline of the car. Looking through the smashed windscreen I found myself face to face with the driver. He was slumped over the steering wheel, or rather where the wheel had been, for it had crumpled and was acting like a spear; I could see a bit of it protruding from his back. He was past the help of anyone. I then heard a feeble groan from deeper inside the car.

No sound or low sound is the worst thing to hear from a patient. If they are making a lot of noise, it generally means they are not too bad; feeble groans mean they have problems. I peered into the car and saw a female crumpled up between the seats. It was about then that I heard loud crashing and was delighted to see three firemen and Pete slipping and sliding down the embankment. The most welcome sight of the day, the cavalry had arrived! Between us we worked out how we could manage to get me, without my coat and tunic, into the car. I stripped off and within seconds my shirt was soaked. It wasn't easy to get into the mangled car even though I was as slim as a post in those days. They sort of held me flat in their arms and fed me in. At last I was inside and taking care not to step on her, I managed to get into a position to carry out an examination on the patient.

She was a young to middle-aged woman, at times like that it's hard to tell. I quickly found a fractured femur and a compound tib and fib. The patient was semi-conscious and had lost a lot of blood from a neck wound. Whilst dressing the wound, I liaised with Pete to get me oxygen, and with the fire crew as to how they were going to get us out. Whilst they are the rescue experts, the patient was my responsibility. We worked out how they could release us, causing the least amount of harm to the patient. I always had a high regard for firemen and none more so than when I was trapped inside a car on a railway track! It is the most important role of an ambulanceman to gain an immediate rapport with the patient. Think about it. You're hurt, in pain, and a strange man starts placing his hands on you! He has to gain your confidence and very quickly. In this case the patient, very fortunately for her, was semi-conscious, this spared her knowledge of a lot of detail. I did my best to ensure her condition remained stable until we could get her out of the car and into hospital, but as I had very little room within the confines of the squashed car, I was limited as to how much I could do.

Whilst I heard everything, I could not see the rescue from my confined space. Luckily a fireman was stationed on the outside and remained with me. He was the link man, and I was pleased to have his company. He told me that the fire crew had tied ropes to a tree and had carried all their equipment down by holding the rope with one hand and sliding down. Anyone who has seen the amount of gear they require to cut open a car will know the task they had. At last the fire crew started to cut the roof off the car. They had to cut carefully and slowly, stopping every few minutes for me to check my patient. I did my best to keep a supply of oxygen to her, and to protect her from the rain dripping in. After what seem an age, the air powered cutter did its task and the top section of roof was lifted off. At last I was able to stand and stretch my cramped limbs. I had been bent double for some time, and it's only when you try to stand up that you realise how cramped you've become. I also discovered it was still pouring with rain and the little protection we had, was now gone. A struggle up and down the embankment by a fireman produced a fire sheet to protect the patient, who fortunately, was still holding her own.

The fire crew were on to the final part of the rescue when Pete's cheerful face appeared at the 'window' in the tarpaulin. He gave his usual big grin and asked "You alright Mate?"

I said I was. The grin got bigger, "I'm pleased about that, and I don't want to worry you, but there's a train here!"

A wave of panic swept through me, surely someone must have told British Rail we were trespassing on one of their lines, and to close it to trains! He laughed for days about my look of panic! In liaison with the Police and Fire, Pete had pointed out we would never get the patient up the embankment. The police said "No problem, we'll get a train to take her out". Another ambulance crew had met

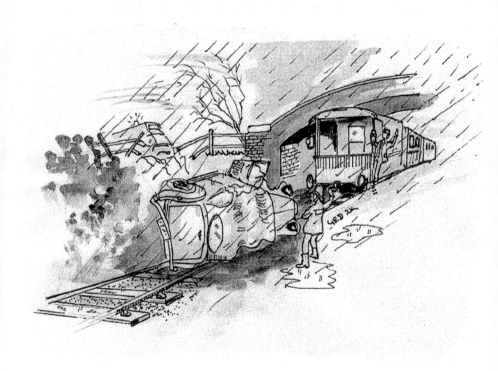

the train at the next station along the line and they brought their equipment along in a guard's van. I must confess I was a little apprehensive to see a large train creeping so close to me, but the plan worked like clockwork. Our patient was loaded onto a stretcher and with a struggle, for a guards van is high from the track, she was transferred to the other crew who took the patient, via train and ambulance to hospital. We were pleased when the police told us they would deal with the deceased driver when released.

It was not without regret that we collected our equipment and with help from the fire crew dragged ourselves up the ropes to the top of the embankment. As you can imagine we were in a terrible condition. The two of us, and all our kit, were wet through and covered in mud. I had lost my cap and Pete a shoe, and although wet and tired we were pleased the rescue had gone as well as it had, demonstrating how well the Emergency Services work together when required.

We climbed wearily into the ambulance and threw our pile of wet, muddy kit and equipment into the back. It was two hours past our finish time, we were both ready for food, bath and bed. Drying my face with a blanket I picked up the radio and told Control we were returning to station. He radioed back at once, could we clear a few outpatients? Restraining ourselves, we politely declined.

CHAPTER SIXTEEN

The Steel Works

The steel works dominated half the town. It dominated life and employment. Steel was the town, not just a piece of history to be talked about by old men gazing into their pints. Steel meant something, it meant work, it meant money. 'Where tha's muck, tha's brass' was a fact of life in that part of the country.

This was the mid 1960's, well before nationalisation, a time when the names of famous steel making companies were known the world over. The works gave employment to thousands, well paid mucky work, but it had little to do with me, I was an ambulanceman, not well paid, and sometimes my job entailed mucky jobs, but in a different sort of way. At least we were mobile and didn't have to go into those horrible dirty and smoky places to work each day. In fact we hardly ever went through the gates, for each company provided its own medical centre and ambulance. We saw them about town and at the hospital but had little or no contact with them. We didn't mind them doing their own thing at all, the rest of the population seemed to find enough work for us to do, being born and everything that could befall them between then and when they died.

We were on the return journey to the station one morning when we received a 'shout' to a steel works. Pete and I looked at each other in amazement as Control passed us the details; we were more than a little surprised for it was indeed a very rare event for us to be called into a works. Neither of us had been into one before, but if they wanted us...

The lights and beacons were switched on and with the horns blaring, off we went. We made good time and arrived at the main gate; a security man met us and, hanging on the running board, escorted us through the site. We bounced past massive buildings, railway lines and trucks, piles of what looked like scrap metal and all sorts of clutter. Everywhere we looked seemed busy, noisy and dirty. At last, totally lost, we reached an enormous corrugated iron building. The escort said it was a 'casting shed', which of course meant absolutely nothing to us. We entered with the stretcher and were taken into the depths of the structure.

It was a vast cathedral of a building. The air was thick with dust, steam and smoke. Weak shafts of sunlight from dirt-encrusted windows high in the distant roof, cut through the haze, highlighting swirling dust clouds which sparkled and danced. The noise was tremendous, with constant hammering, crashing and clanging. Dante's *Inferno* must be something like this. As we went deeper into the depths of the building we became very aware of the intense heat and the reason for this quickly became apparent. Continuous lengths of red hot steel wound their way around rollers and channels in the floor. At times we found ourselves only feet away from the molten metal and watched fascinated, and a little scared, as we followed our guide. At last, at the centre of the building he stopped, and we found we had arrived at the scene of the incident. At the base of a large machine was a group of men and a body. We could tell it was a 'body' as opposed to a 'patient' because the head was missing. As with most incidents, the group of workmen stood around doing nothing. They watched us and said nothing, just awaiting our arrival. A big burly man, who must have been the foreman, stepped forward and asked us to remove the body. Although he didn't say it, I had the distinct feeling the request was occasioned by halted production rather than compassion.

I asked what had happened before either of us handled the body, well aware that if there was any chance of foul play, the police would not want anything touched. Two men started to tell us, but a look from the big man silenced them, and we realised at once from his look that he was the boss and it was obviously his job to explain. He seemed to relish his position of power and began to slowly give us the background information of the events that had lead to this death. His size and bulk did not make us inclined to interrupt.

The casualty had been a sweeper-up. Those were the days of full employment, and although it may seem hard to believe now, there were more jobs than workers. A sweeper-up in a steel works did not earn a lot and the applicants were generally not of the highest quality, and employers took what they could get. Someone said afterwards it was a bit like the Ambulance Service taking me on! This man had been what could be called 'not all there' or 'none too sharp' – one of life's misfits. It seemed he would wander around the building all day leaning on his brush, pushing the waste around until it fell off, not achieving much but in his own simple way 'doing his bit'.

We learned that the machine he was under was an enormous guillotine of some tons, this chopped the newly formed steel into short lengths which in time became nails or cars or something. It would seem that this poor soul would spend ages looking at the guillotine every day as he passed, leaning on his brush, his head going up and down in time with the guillotine's action. It was clear the machine fascinated him. We surmised that his curiosity had got the better of him on that particular morning and he must have put his head under it to see it from a new angle! When, at long last the big man stopped talking I looked around, and asked the important question, "Where's his head?" Someone pointed it out to me, lying some way down the aisle in a gutter. I asked them to fetch it over but received the response from the big man.

"Tha's the bloody ambulanceman you ger it!"

Which was just what I did. Like all crowds who gather to watch an accident, they didn't want to miss anything but also they didn't want to touch.

We loaded the body onto the stretcher after I had retrieved the head. At this point, experience came into play. There was no point in putting the head on to the pillow for it would fall off, so, the safest place was between the deceased legs where there was no chance of us losing it. We covered the body with a blanket, and were rather surprised to discover that no one was going to accompany us to the hospital. The foreman said that 'Medical' would sort it out.

So off we went with our guide back through the murk to find our ambulance. Having loaded, and whilst Pete was finding his way out of the maze of roads in the works, I radioed to Control and informed them we were leaving for the hospital with a suspected DOA (dead on arrival) and would they please inform the hospital. In those days an ambulanceman could not pronounce death, hence the term 'suspected'. Control then telephoned the A&E department and told them we were on the way with a suspected BID (brought in dead). Note the change in designation, NHS jargon, but still 'suspected'.

Arriving at the hospital we drove to the back doors of the A&E department, I went inside to find the Doctor whilst Pete stayed with the patient. At this point I should perhaps explain procedures. Every hospital patient must be accompanied by records, a very fair point, as this gives the hospital a chance of knowing what is happening and who is inside the building. Whilst an ambulanceman could not pronounce death, if he thought that was the case, a Doctor would examine the patient in the ambulance and certify death. Thus the patient would not go on record as having died in the A&E Department. So when newspapers say '... was found to be dead on arrival at hospital' it does not mean, as most people seem to think, that they died in the ambulance. I would hasten to add that this is only in cases when life is obviously extinct – if there is any chance of life then everything possible is done to save the patient.

I met the Doctor and together with a Sister he came outside with me. Opening the rear door of the ambulance, I helped them in. Now, at this point, please don't think I am being critical of other people's abilities. I would never make any criticism of a Junior Hospital Doctor, they have a terrible time, long hours, rotten shifts, and are at the beck and call of everyone. They are blamed by the patients for delays, poor treatment, draughts, canteen tea, pages missing from magazines and whatever political party is in office. These young doctors have my every sympathy, so when this gentleman pulled back the blanket, put his stethoscope on the patient's chest and shut his eyes, it was not for me to say anything, after all he was the Doctor, and me a simple ambulanceman. I expect the poor guy had been on duty since the night before.

I may have said nothing, but not so the Sister.

"Doctor you don't need that…" she boomed, in a voice loud enough to jolt him back to reality.

The Doctor scowled at the Sister and then glanced down at the headless corpse. A look of shock came on his face, he then gave a horrified yelp and departed quickly, shouting at me in a strange foreign tongue. Sister stood her ground and asked me where the head was. With a flourish I removed the blanket to reveal the face of the deceased looking at her from between his legs. Being a practical and compassionate woman, Sister announced I couldn't leave the head in that position and she would provide a receptacle for it. She returned a short time later with a plastic bag from a well known grocery chain, into which we put the head of the deceased. Saying 'you know what to do' the Sister left us. From this I made the assumption that the Doctor's words when he had left hurriedly indicated he had pronounced death and the body could now be removed to the mortuary, which, like every hospital mortuary, was in the hospital grounds tucked out of sight, away from public view.

If a body had been found in anything like suspicious circumstances, the police had to be informed immediately. They would then arrange for an officer to be at the morgue to accept the body when we arrived. Again there was an established procedure, a radio call would be made to Ambulance Control, who would inform the police. This done, off we would go. We had been told this enabled the police to have the nearest PC awaiting us. Pull the other one! I will never be anything but convinced that when they received a message like that, they scoured the town to find the newest copper they had, and then sent that poor sod!

Naturally, when we arrived at the morgue there was no one in sight, neither police nor porter. As we had little emergency cover in those days, we didn't bother to waste time waiting, and started to unload. We knew the procedure well enough and what was required. Taking the body off the ambulance we placed it onto a trolley, found a vacant compartment in the huge fridge, and placed the corpse inside. It was at this point, as we were almost finished, that a face appeared around the edge of the door. A very pale face; a very young pale face; very worried and hardly visible beneath an oversized helmet. The helmet appeared to be too large for one so young, almost like a child playing with something belonging to his father. Furthermore, the helmet appeared to be supported mainly by his ears, which were large and very prominent. Our policeman looked extremely young and very new, I would guess about fourteen years old! It stood out a mile he was just out of training school, it must have been his first day on the streets alone and I guessed it was his first visit to a morgue. The law had again acted true to form!

I smiled at the lad, trying to re-assure him.

"You can come in, we've put him in the fridge out of sight, it's all done and he's all yours."

The policeman looked very relieved and entered the room, pulling up his big gloves. Now fully in control, he was in charge, his whole attitude had become one of, I'm the copper, I'm in charge, out of my way you mere ambulanceman. The policeman's change of attitude immediately put my back up. I stood waiting for him, beginning to fume at his newly found courage. Usually we got on well with the law, but I didn't feel inclined to be bossed about by a cocky kid. Then it came to me. In my hand I held a plastic bag, a bag from a well known grocery chain! I wouldn't have thought about doing it if he hadn't become so arrogant. From being a timid young boy who needed help and protection he had tried to become the hard copper. His words had my hackles up.

"OK, I'll look after things now, you lot clear off," thus dismissing us from his thoughts. Obviously, a mere ambulanceman was beneath him, not worth the effort of conversing with. Now he had really rubbed me up the wrong way. By now, I was really fuming.

It was wrong, I knew it was wrong, it did not show respect for the dead nor was it professional, but I had to do it, I couldn't resist. With a straight face and avoiding the look of horror on the face of my mate standing behind him, I held out the bag to the Constable. "You had better take this, you'll need it." The Police Constable reached for the bag.

"Is it his?" he grunted indicating the body he had not seen. I nodded. Again the man gave a dismissive nod of the head. We didn't wait to see him open the bag. As one, Pete and I bolted out of the door and into our vehicle. Pete, almost choking with suppressed chuckles and excitement started the engine and it roared into life. We took off in a cloud of blue exhaust smoke. Over the powerful roar of the big six cylinder Bedford engine we heard a scream of horror.

We were very careful where we parked our cars for the next few weeks.

CHAPTER SEVENTEEN

Risk to Life and Limb

Everyone knows that fire crews risk their lives at fires, and the policeman on the beat comes across dangerous situations, but most people think that ambulance crews have a pretty safe job. In and out of houses and hospitals, drinking tea. However, you may not think so but it can be pretty hairy at times believe me.

No matter what we were doing, the sudden clanging of the emergency bell would always send blood racing and hearts pounding, adrenaline surging. Whoever decided to install that large and powerful bell had obviously never been nearby when it had gone off.

It was a beautiful hot Saturday afternoon, one of those very occasional hot days when all you want to do is sink into a pool or to go to sleep in the sun. We'd had a busy morning and were enjoying a cuppa after lunch, enjoying the warmth of the sun on us as we sat outside the office. I am sure we were both at that point between day dreaming and nodding off when the damn bell above our heads crashed into action. You have to experience a noise like that to know how it affects you. I am sure that is the reason why you never meet a lot of old ambulancemen! Of course you never had time to think about it when it happened, it was a mad scramble to grab caps, kit and sprint to the ambulance, a cross between a Le Mans start and a scramble to a Spitfire during the Battle of Britain. I leapt into the driving seat and gunned the engine into life whilst Pete called Control. The detail was to a local brewery, a man in a vat of beer, Fire Crew attending.

Pete chuckled. "I'll go back and get me mug, we can have a party!"

With horns blaring and lights blazing we swung out of the station yard. Luckily for us the local team were playing away that weekend, had it have been a home match day we would have experienced problems attempting to get to the part of town where the accident had taken place. As it was, the roads were crowded. Whenever we went on an emergency I was sure I came across a rally of the CHARD club (our name for confused, half asleep and retarded drivers). I don't wish to cast aspersions against the great British driving public, but it never ceased to amaze me how drivers could manage to not see or hear a large white ambulance with lights blazing and klaxons screaming. Most people were sensible and kept an eye on the road ahead and the rear view mirror, they saw us and got out of the way. The remainder, a minority, seemed to be divided between those who didn't see us and those who didn't care. As we sped down the road it was routine to 'drive ahead' to watch traffic flow and anticipate what could happen before it did. Most cars would pull into the side as they saw us coming but we soon learned to spot well in advance the ones who were oblivious to us. When those drivers at last got the message they would do one of two things, jump on the brakes and stop in the middle of the road, thus blocking our path, or try to race us. Whatever happened, we had to get ahead of them one way or the other. The very factor of manoeuvring a large vehicle at speed, in a crowded town could and did give us a few hairy moments.

Despite all the usual problems, we made good time to the brewery and could smell it as soon as we swung into the main gates. A very excited and panicking gateman met us and pointed to a building where another man frantically beckoned. We followed our guide into the depths of the building and started to climb steps and fixed ladders ever upward as we proceeded to the upper reaches of the barn-like building.

Every part seemed to consist of shiny steel pipes going in all directions to valves and gauges, all between polished steel walls. It was not until we reached the top of one of the gantries that we discovered the steel walls were, in fact, enormous vats containing fermenting beer. The top of one of the vats was open, and we saw that the surface of the liquid was covered in a deep crust of dark brown bubbles and sludge. It looked horrible, enough to put you off drinking for good. But among this foul substance we caught sight of a man in the centre. He was, of course, covered in the stuff, laying across and hanging on to the end of a ladder which was being held at the other end by three men. At first I couldn't understand why they had not pulled him in to safety, but quickly discovered that his leg was caught in a paddle like thing that mixed up the fermenting liquid. Every time they tried to pull him in he screamed in pain. At that point we were both pleased to hear the sound of more two-tone horns which announced the arrival of the Fire Service; we were well aware we needed their expertise on this one.

We could see that the patient was in a lot of pain and getting weaker. He was also moving rapidly into a state of shock. The fire crew arrived and we conferred with the sub-officer. Although it was a large building, everywhere was full of brewing equipment with very little room to work. Whilst a plan for getting the man out was devised, the fire crew took over from the workers and held the ladder supporting the patient. It was plain that in addition to everything else, the heavy fumes from the fermenting beer were having a noticeable effect on him. We too were also beginning to feel its effects. The fire lads worked out a plan using ladders and lengths of wood to reach the patient, having found out it would be impractical to empty the vat. Whilst this was going on Pete and I were getting concerned about the patient. We had to get oxygen to him or the rescue was going to be of no use for he was soon going to pass out and drop into the liquid. The Sub said that they would get a supporting ladder, so that someone could lie on it and crawl to him. Pete and I looked at each other, the same thought in our minds. The patient was our responsibility, despite the offer of the fire crew, it was our job to deal with him. It was also plain to see that I was the lightest of the two of us.

The fire crew looked after me well, they tied two ropes around me, in case I fell in, and rigged up a second ladder. Although they assured me it was safe, it didn't look it. I was not into this Commando sort of thing! I was scared stiff. They tried to reassure me that their contraption was safe but I didn't believe them. Clutching the oxygen set tightly, and feeling the ropes taut around me on each side, I inched along the ladder. It's not an easy thing to shuffle along a flat ladder with one hand whilst the other is clasping an oxygen set. It was also not helped by the sight of all that gunge so close below and knowing it was very deep. I was convinced the stuff was waiting for me and looking forward to gobbling me up. Funny the way the mind works when you're scared!

After what seemed an age, and soaked with a mixture of sweat and beer, I reached the patient. He needed the oxygen badly. We lay together clutching each other like long lost brothers. I held the mask against the man's face. The smell of the fermenting beer was overpowering and every now and again I had to take the mask to have a lung full of the oxygen to keep myself conscious. All the time I could hear the fire crew working frantically to make good the rescue and shouting reassuring words to me. However, as I lay there, I became aware that our combined weight was causing the support to sink into the liquid. Panic set in! I didn't dare tell my patient and hoped my concern didn't show. I had safety ropes on me but I had never been so scared in my life.

As the oxygen brought him round, and my presence and sight of the fire crew gave him reassurance, the patient began to talk to me. As he did, I managed, inch by inch, to move alongside of him until I could check his legs. At last I discovered his leg was not broken as we had feared, but realised he was trapped by his boot. Almost frightening myself to death, as we clung to each other, I somehow managed to get his foot free. He was no longer trapped! Pete told me later that my shout of "Ger us in!" was almost a scream, and I believe him.

The fire lads had almost completed their plan and in no time I felt our ladder and the ropes start to move. I know they did a fantastic job, but the return journey out of the vat seemed the longest period of time in my life. I've never been so pleased to feel hands on me. In no time we were on firm ground. Pete and the fire crew made the patient comfortable and got him down to the ambulance. I couldn't stop shaking, I had to rest and calm down before a fireman helped me down to the ground.

I was exhausted, mentally and physically, so Pete and the firemen loaded the patient into the ambulance. As I was in no fit state to do anything, I was pushed into the back with the patient and Pete drove us to the hospital. Luckily the A&E department was only a short distance away and in no time the patient was helped in. By then, I had stopped shaking to some degree and was beginning to feel a little more human. Sister insisted the duty doctor check me over, and the whole of the department seemed to come in to see me. After an examination by the doctor I was pronounced fit and he gave me a couple of aspirins, saying I'd be fine. I felt he had more confidence in me than I had. We climbed back into the ambulance and explained our situation to Control. We then returned to station via my home, for I had to change. When my wife saw me, her nose wrinkled in disgust.

"Where on earth have you been? You smell just like a boozer..." That was all I needed!

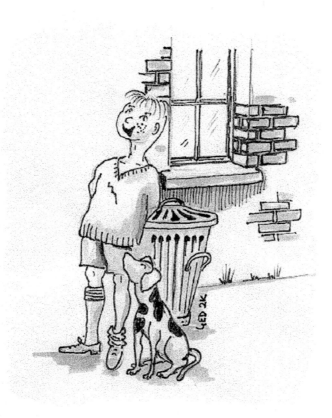

CHAPTER EIGHTEEN

The Faux-Pas

The raucous blast of klaxon horns echoed back from ranks of terraced houses in the narrow streets. Twin blue beacons on the ambulance roof created crazy reflections and flashes of light in passing windows. Pete's hands and feet moved non stop as he controlled the big Bedford ambulance, weaving around parked cars forcing oncoming traffic onto the pavements. It was the second emergency of the shift and we'd only been on duty an hour, our newly scrounged cups of tea still hot on Sister's desk in the casualty department. It looked as though we were in for a busy night.

The call was a collapse case; it was too early for drunks and far too late for shoppers, so this could be a real emergency.

The narrow streets of this part of town had been built for steel workers in the latter days of the nineteenth century, long before the invention of cars. Although it was supposed to be the poorer end of town, the number of parked cars made you wonder if the welfare state was as bad as the media constantly claimed. A ramshackle black and rust Ford pulled into what the youthful driver obviously thought was near enough to the side of the road. Pete swore and skilfully took our big J2 through the gap at speed with inches to spare. I trusted Pete's driving, but a quick glance at the look of horror on the spotty face of the youth made me think he had a number of doubts. I couldn't help but notice that his girlfriend was a cracking bit of stuff. As Pete swung us into the street of the call-out, I reached across to flick off horns and beacons. The size of the ambulance would attract the inevitable onlookers quickly enough without providing music and illumination to attract more and provide entertainment. I called Control by RT and told them we were 'on scene'. Pete double parked; he had no option. One advantage of an ambulance on an emergency, no one complains about you blocking the road. Whilst I went over to the house with the emergency case and blanket, Pete opened the back doors and ensured all was ready for the patient before coming to join me.

It was a typical town street where the houses opened directly onto the pavement. Outside number 38, a policewoman knelt with her face to the letter box talking to someone inside. Two portly women in the inevitable curlers, head scarves and cross-over pinnies stood, with arms folded, offering advice and guidance to the young constable. Like all professionals in that type of situation, she ignored them. At least a dozen scruffy kids had gathered around to pass the time of day and watch the fun. I squeezed through the seething mass, ignoring the plaintive cry from a two foot tall potential troublemaker, clasping a football.

"Oo the 'ell der yer fink yer pushin?" he sniffed.

I knelt beside the policewoman. She looked across at me and smiled with obvious relief saying she was pleased to see us. Experience had taught me that, whilst the police went out of their way to help us at all times, they were the first to admit to being pleased to see an ambulance at an incident involving casualties. It was very noticeable, and appreciated, how they would step back and let us take over. A good relationship existed between the two services; an unwritten rule of each to his own. I wholeheartedly agreed with this and always made a point of letting a copper go into a punch-up first!

The policewoman swiftly explained that the occupier, a Mrs Jackson, an old lady, lived alone and had fallen, jamming herself against the door. Mrs Jackson was conscious but could not move. At that point, one of the women watching the action must have thought I was most probably deaf for she repeated the policewoman's message, word for word. I put my mouth to the letterbox and spoke to the patient. One of the rules of our job is 'never accept the word of anyone regarding a patient if you can check it for yourself'. The old lady assured me she was in good spirits and although not in pain, could not move away from the door or reach up to open it. Like all old people of her generation Mrs Jackson apologised over and over again for being any trouble. At that point, one of the watching women started to tell me the life history of the patient. By the time she had reached Emily Jackson's marriage, I pointedly suggested she went to make us all a cup of tea. The woman may have looked rough and stupid but she wasn't going to make tea and miss the best bit of excitement on the street for weeks. We now had a problem of getting to our patient. The easy way was to smash the front window; not the glass in the door, for that could drop onto the patient and cause more injury to her. But we were well aware that, no matter what we said to Mrs Jackson, as an old person she would worry if we broke any glass in the house. I decided that, as the patient was conscious and had assured me she was not in pain nor bleeding, the best alternative was to send for help. Help in the form of the Fire Brigade. The fire lads would have the door off in a flash. Pete quickly agreed and returned the radio to request their attendance.

Meanwhile we were stuck, with the patient happily talking to the policewoman through the door. While we were waiting, I thought I'd have a look around the back of the house to see if there was any other way I could get in. I explained my intention to the policewoman and Pete, left them with the patient and forced my way through the crowd of onlookers, which had now grown to epic proportions – I would not have been at all surprised to have seen bus-loads more spectators arrive at any moment.

Counting the houses carefully, I walked along the terrace until reaching the end of the street, then made my way along the side of the block to the cobbled alley which ran behind the houses, separating them from the backs of those in the next street. Counting again, I stopped at the back of the house and surveyed my problem. At this point a small voice piped up behind me.

"Wot yer gonna do mista?"

I looked down and in the rapidly gathering gloom saw the small figure that had joined me in the otherwise deserted alley. The boy was about five years old and looked as though he was about to audition for a part in Oliver, or perhaps he was a model for *Viz* or *The Beano*. His ragged jersey was many sizes too large for his skinny frame and in the centre of his chest was a large rip through which could be seen a grubby grey school shirt. In contrast, his shorts were too tight, exposing a length of spindly leg, one grey sock up and the other crumpled around his ankle; both knees were grubby and scratched. The lad's mousy hair looked as though it had been cut around a basin. I then noticed a rather nondescript black and white mongrel dog by his side, head cocked to one side looking up at me. The dog was studying me, guessing correctly that I was not one of its own tribe. I smiled down at the boy, and then looked at the back of the house.

Success! I spotted the upper section of a ground floor window was open. I decided I could just about manage to get through that window with a struggle. My plan of action was rudely interrupted as I felt a tug at the bottom of my raincoat.

"Eh-up, ah said wot's thee gona do mista. Dint thee ere me?"

I smiled down at the lad, feeling sorry for him.

"I'm going to climb through that window and go to help the old lady in number 38." The boy looked up at me with wonder in his eyes. Huge dark eyes filled with experience, clearly wise beyond his tender age. He eyed me up and down, then with a scowl looked up and stared hard at the tiny window. His gaze dropped down at his dog which cocked its head to the other side and seemed to smile up at him. The boy gave a deep sigh and shaking his head returned his attention back to me. That little chap looked quite angelic as he spoke.

"Bagger orf yer silly owd sod. Tha's far too friggin owd 'n fat ter ger in there."

With this pronouncement the boy turned and ran back down the alley as fast as those spindly legs would carry him. The silent alley echoed with shrieks of high pitched laughter. The dog bounded by his side barking excitedly, I was sure that dog was laughing at me as well.

Shedding raincoat and tunic I dragged a handy dustbin over to the window and stepped up on to it. With a loud clatter the lid shot from under foot and my leg rammed into the foul smelling contents. I swore and started again. With a lot of struggling and effort, delighted the boy had left me, I managed to work my way through the window. Too old and fat, cheeky little sod. I almost fell into the bathroom, knocking over a tin of talc which went everywhere, including over me. As I lay panting on the floor I reached the decision that maybe, just maybe, I was out of condition and would never make a burglar.

After what seemed an age I regained my breath and managed to struggle to my feet. Knowing the layout of this type of house I went through into the kitchen. It was very surprising how modern and well equipped the room was for an old lady, most unusual. I then made my way into the passage leading to the front door and was amazed to find a wall stopping me reaching my patient. Horror and panic surged through me. It dawned on me that the house had been converted into two flats and I was in the wrong one! Was I about to bump into another old lady and give her a heart attack? Was I about to be attacked by a big dog? Maybe meet a big man with a stick thinking he had caught a burglar? Or a young lady in the nude? Even that thought frightened me! Fortunately, the house was silent and empty. I let myself out of the kitchen door, grabbed my gear from among the spilt refuse and ran.

Arriving back at the front of the house I paused to regain my breath. Forcing my way through the crowd I was delighted to find Pete and a police car crew had managed to get the door open to reach the old lady. Better still she was none the worse for her ordeal. Pete looked quizzically at me, pulling a face as we put Mrs Jackson onto the stretcher and loaded her into the ambulance. We were all pleased to be out of sight of our now considerable audience, me even more so. I asked a copper to step into the ambulance with me and made a rather shamefaced explanation of my faux-pas. To my relief and growing embarrassment, the copper roared with laughter. Clearly he though it a great joke. As his mirth subsided, he did, however, promise to make amends to the householder and sort out any problems. Just as Pete was closing the back doors on us I cringed, recognising a plaintive shrill voice.

"Towed yer the owd sod was too friggin owd n fat ter ger in the 'ouse!"

The hairs on the back of my neck bristled. I pretended not to hear.

CHAPTER NINETEEN

The Ambulance Drove Away

'When the bells go down' had a distinct meaning in those far-off days. Both inside the crew room and outside in the yard the enormous bells indicated an emergency by a ten second ring. Ten seconds may not sound a long time but in those situations it was enough to waken the dead and frighten the life out of us.

Pete and I had booked on duty for a late shift, three until eleven. Since the introduction of regular partners, we had become a good team. If you had a good mate you were happy, a bad one and you applied for the first available shift change. We worked well together, taking turns to drive or to be attendant. Each knew what the other was going to do in either role, it was a bit like a marriage. Every crew followed the same procedure as soon as they got on station for their shift. The driver checked the mechanics and the exterior of the vehicle, the attendant checked the interior and ambulance equipment. It didn't matter if the ambulance had not been out, it was your job to make sure all was where it should be for someone's life could depend upon it. In the interior, each piece of equipment had a storage place and it had to be ready for immediate use. Gas cylinders had to be full or changed and any kit used had to be replaced. In winter, a hot water bottle would go between the blankets. The driver ensured all levels were correct, the tank full of petrol and the emergency warning devices functioning. As the weather was fine that day we followed our usual procedure and drove the bus across the yard, parking next to the crew room. We always parked with the bonnet pointing at the gate ready to go. As a radio check had informed Control we were on duty, we again followed the usual procedure and made a cup of tea.

It was a funny thing about tea, as I have said before, you never refused a cup, be it on station, hospital department or anywhere. You never knew if you would have time to finish it or, more to the point, when you'd get the chance of another one. We always felt sure there was a secret indicator that made the emergency call come in just as you poured the water into the pot!

This time it was an unusually quiet shift, nothing happened, nothing at all. In fact at about five we settled down in front of the TV and had our sandwiches, and of course, a pot of tea. Crews came in and left for their homes. By six o'clock everyone had gone home and we were left alone. We decided to watch the news and then start on the range of chores undertaken by the late shift crew. The peace was suddenly broken as the bells went off. The raucous clanging vibrated around the small room, changing the scene of laid-back peace and tranquillity to one of controlled and urgent action. As one, we were out of the door grabbing caps and struggling into tunics. Pete started the motor and revved hard to warm it up in the quickest time. Ambulances were used to going from cold to maximum revs in no time, it always seemed to work and they never let us down... but never buy a second hand ambulance!

Meanwhile I had grabbed my first aid case from the porch and leapt into the attendant's seat radioing in for details. Pete had the Bedford rolling towards the gates, waiting to hear the location of the job to know whether he should turn right or left. Control informed us it was a Road Traffic Accident on the High Street, only a quarter of a mile from the station. As soon as the location came through, Pete put his foot down and simultaneously switched on headlights and beacon. I put my foot on the horn switch and kept it there. The ambulance leapt forward, swinging into the street and roaring off towards our destination.

We were so close to the incident that bystanders would hear us coming immediately. As the ambulance turned into the main road we saw a knot of people and a figure laid on the ground. I radioed in to tell control we were 'on scene'. As Pete pulled up at the accident, I jumped out and went to the patient. We always followed the same procedure, regardless of who was 'driver' or 'attendant'. The attendant went to the scene whilst the driver weighed up whether back-up was required. He would then park the ambulance facing the direction we intended to leave the scene and in a position that would protect the patient and ourselves. This procedure was essential, for motorists seemed to have little regard for ambulancemen, and in addition, in those days we were dressed in navy blue, no one had thought of high-visibility clothing, and at night we were well aware that we were at high risk.

I pushed my way through the crowd of onlookers and knelt down by the patient. He was a young man of about 25 who told me he had skidded on a manhole cover and fallen off his bike. He had received a bang on his head and a nasty case of gravel rash down the side of his face with abrasions to his hand and arm. Nothing serious. He assured me he had not been unconscious and remembered everything. I was applying a dressing to his face when a voice from the crowd asked me where my mate was going. I didn't look up and said over my shoulder that he was positioning the ambulance for the hospital.

After a pause the voice spoke again and asked was I sure? I had long ceased to become annoyed when bystanders asked silly questions at an incident, even when, as in this case, no one had done anything to help the patient before we arrived. I looked up, about to make a sarcastic comment, and froze. He was right! Pete and the ambulance had gone! Disappeared. Not a sign. Hells bells! This was new to me. I had experienced a number of things during my service but this was something I had never come across before. Had I said something to upset Pete? I experienced a moment of panic! I forced myself to think. Experience had taught me a lot. It had taught me how to deal with patients and people; it had also taught me that people panic very easily. If I gave the impression that all was not right it could create problems, not only for the patient but also me! So I decided to do what I was good at and look after the patient. I found another bandage and started to chat to him.

"Ere, why's yer mate cleared orf?". The voice was becoming shrill, echoing the panic I was now beginning to feel. I was also getting annoyed, it was my job to panic, nothing to do with him.

"Sod off," I muttered under my breath.

I looked up at the scrawny figure scowling down at me and smiled reassuringly. "He's positioning the ambulance for me," I explained, hoping I gave the impression of knowing what was happening. I for one did not believe this! The skinny prat must have been a member of the local dramatic society, for he put his hand up above his eyes, screwing them up to give the impression he was searching the ocean. He slowly moved slowly around well aware he was receiving everyone's attention.

"I can't see owt, 'ees positioned well!"

I could have hit the silly sod, but I managed to restrain myself. Just then a female voice said, "Shut up clot, let the chap get on with it. He knows what he's doing"

I smiled up at the portly lady and thanked her, pleased I still had the sensible ones on my side.

But where the hell was Pete! I worked on pretending to concentrate on what I was doing so that no one could see my face.

"There you are! I said he knew what they were doing," the same female voice announced. With that, the gleaming white ambulance pulled up alongside me and Pete leapt out. Within moments the stretcher was placed by my side and in no time we had our patient loaded into the back of the ambulance. The doors slammed and I felt relief flood over me as we pulled away. It was only a short run into casualty, my patient chatted about everything and nothing, not noticing anything had gone wrong. I was most relieved he'd not been badly injured. Very soon the patient was transferred into the care of a nurse in the department. Once outside the doors my relief turned to anger.

"What's the chuffing game, leaving me in the middle of the High Street whilst you clear off for a tour of the town?"

My burst of temper was not helped when Pete burst out laughing. Within moments he literally rolled, tears running down his cheeks, almost choking, banging his fists against the ambulance. He had one of those infectious sort of laughs that make you join in. Very soon we were both rolling together like two silly schoolboys, laughing until tears ran down our cheeks. The silly thing was I didn't know why I was laughing! At last we settled down and Pete explained what had happened. Having parked at the incident he'd opened the back doors to find the interior bare. Not a thing inside the ambulance – empty! As we were so near the station he did not bother to tell me but returned and discovered what had happened.

The ambulance we had taken in our haste had been returned from major service by the workshop fitters, who, not thinking, had parked it between the crew room and our waiting vehicle. One white Bedford looks much like the next, and as we never thought to look in the back and as we always left the keys in the ignition it never occurred to us it may not have been the right ambulance. But suppose the accident had been well out of town, or a bad one! I still feel a chill at the thought of what might have happened!

CHAPTER TWENTY

Promotion

It was Alan Barker who started it all. If he hadn't said anything I'd still have been there, still have been an ambulanceman looking forward to retiring. Like most things in life that have had a profound effect upon me, it started as a joke.

Pete was on leave and I was on a funny part of the rota, one of those weeks where you were the odd bod on station, a bit like a spare thing at a wedding. You took sitting outpatients on long runs, you transferred vehicles, you helped in the office, you ran about, made tea, counted the pencils and generally acted as a runner, you were, in every sense of the word the 'gofer'.

The new system had settled down and Alan was proving his worth as Station Officer. Alan was a guy who put staff, patients and the Service all to the forefront of his life. Never in a thousand years could he be compared to Godly in looks, actions or temperament. You could talk to him and learn. That afternoon he had been to a meeting and in his absence I, at a loose end, had sat at his desk and started to collate a few figures on his statistical returns. I was quite enjoying it, it was a change from my normal role. Someone from HQ Admin had rung and I had taken a list of information from her. I was laid back in the chair chatting to her when Alan came in. He indicated to me to continue and busied himself at the other desk. After I had finished he remarked how I looked the part at a desk, and asked why I had never applied for promotion. The thought had never crossed my mind. The two L/A posts on the station had been removed, and in any case, I related Leading Hands to Noddy and Flapper.

Alan told me there was shortly to be a vacancy at a sub station and asked why I didn't apply for it. I scoffed at the idea, me as a Leading Ambulanceman. And leave my home town? Never!

But he had put a seed into my mind and it began to germinate. The more I thought about it, the more it began to appeal to me. I was to learn many times during my career that the promotion bug is one of the most infectious. The Service comprised of a number of main stations located around the county, each manned 24 hours a day, similar to the one I was on. In addition there were four small sub-stations in market towns, each run by a Leading Hand who was responsible to a main station. The man in charge of one not too far from us had been promoted to Control, so his job was up for grabs. I began to think and began to make a few discreet enquiries. That weekend I suggested to my wife that perhaps we should have a ride out into the country, give the kids a change! It was a town we'd never been to before. I had driven through it but never noticed anything. This time the town did seem to be a nice little place, one main street with an assortment of shops and pubs, not unlike most small English market towns. I was about to turn round and run through it again when my wife said, "When does it start?" I had to confess it had started and finished. As one brought up in a big town and used to a range of facilities she was not impressed.

The more I thought about promotion the more the bug gnawed. I persuaded my wife it would be a fantastic place for the kids to grow up, lots of green fields and woods for them to explore. I also pointed out it was only an hours drive back to our old home area. At last she said yes, and I requested an application form for the post. Well that was what I thought would happen, but it didn't quite work out like that. I had expected an advertisement and application forms but found I had to write a letter expressing an interest. I did as requested, listing all the reasons why I considered I was the best man for the job and waited for a reply, and waited, and waited. Weeks went by and still I heard nothing. I thought the letter had been lost and kept nagging Alan. He explained each time I got at him that, as all appointments had to be agreed by the Council, and they only met now and again, it was a slow old job. This was all very well but no use to me, I wanted that promotion, I wanted to go. Now! I learned later that when the Council had at last agreed to fill the post, my application had caused some concern at HQ. It was the only one! Of the two full-timers at the station one had said he wanted the job and the other had said no thank you. So it would have been an easy choice had I not have applied and upset the established routine.

In those days, no one dreamt of moving stations. A job of L/A at a small sub-station involving a pay increase of seven and a half percent, was not even considered by anyone. Apart from this and all other factors involved, the

Council did not pay any removal expenses. The fact that one idiot had elected to apply, which would necessitate a move, gave them food for thought. I learned that the CAO was enthusiastic about my application and as a result advertised the post throughout the Service, an unheard of occurrence. Needless to say no one, apart from Bert and I applied. By now Bert, who was the sitting tenant so to speak, was moaning why was he not being given the job as it was his turn. The CAO decided to come to see me. I was still new to the Service, and furthermore, my army background made me circumspect of rank badges. To be requested to come into station to see the Chief gave me cause for great concern. I was very wary as I entered the station and shown in to the office to see the Chief sitting behind the desk resplendent in his uniform. Well, he must have thought he looked good. He was a fantastic guy, one of the best bosses I ever had but, but he was not designed to wear a uniform, and the uniform was not designed for him!

His uniform proved the point that the Council did not consider its Chief Ambulance Officer required any better tailoring than the rest of us. It was cut in a better style, in a better material and the chrome rank badges decorating it made it look better, but it didn't fit. His shape would have been a challenge to Saville Row and it had beaten the Council's tailor hands down! The tunic seemed to hang on him as though he had left the coat hanger in it. Wherever it stopped, long bits of him stuck out. His sleeves seemed to stop at his elbows and his neck emerged out of the top like a cartoon character. The trousers gave up the struggle three quarters of the way down his spindly legs about mid calf, exposing a length of white leg above his sock. In the whole of my service I never met anyone who could look so out of place in a uniform, or understood how anyone could make clothes look so bad. That apart, he grilled me. Between the "Luk hue" and "Boy-O's" he asked me non stop questions. In no time he knew more about me and my potential and aspirations than I did. He announced that he would interview Bert and I and select the best. I spent a lot of time seeking information regarding what I thought would be required of the post, and learning interview techniques. Although I had no idea at the time, Bert made no effort. On the day of the interview I was full of knowledge, my uniform was immaculate, my boots were bulled, I was full of confidence. That was until I met the dog!

To ensure nothing went wrong I had taken a day's leave. I had arrived at HQ with an hour to spare, just to make sure, and to be able to wind down and be ready for the interview. I sat in the rest room looking at my notes and was horrified when an L/A came in and said we had an emergency.

"Don't worry kid they know what you are doing, they'll wait, and it will look good for you!"

I didn't believe him, but feeling I had no choice I reluctantly went with him. He drove, for I had no idea of the layout of the town. All the time as he weaved in and out of the traffic at speed he kept up a non-stop conversation. Told me not to worry as Bert, my opposition, hadn't a chance. Later when I got to know Bert I was to find the L/A had been right, but it was no consolation that afternoon. We sped to one of the more scruffy areas of town, and pulled up outside what must have been one of the more scruffy houses! I followed the L/A in through the open door into the back room of the house. There we found a man collapsed, obviously the worse for drink. The room smelt of dogs, stale beer and urine. The curtains were drawn, it was dark and filthy. A very large and nondescript mongrel eyed us and constantly growled from its bed, which was an old army blanket on the floor in the corner. An old woman, clasping a mug of tea, sat in a scruffy and grease stained arm chair and kept shouting "Shurrup!" She did not seem greatly interested in the old man on the floor. The dog kept growling.

I was aware as soon as I knelt in the gloom beside the patient that I had put my knee in a pool of urine. As if that was not enough, a moment later the patient rolled over and proceeded to vomit into my upturned cap! We checked his airway and gave him oxygen. At the moment the patient stopped breathing the Doctor arrived. The three of us at once started to work, the L/A with oxygen, the doctor gave an injection and I gave cardiac massage. We worked on that patient long enough for me to start to sweat before he started to respond to us. As I rocked on my heels doing CPR I felt the dog by my side sniffing my shoulder. I was rather relived when it wandered over to the doctor and started to lick his ear. At least it was not going to bite me. The doctor was not afraid of the dog and shouted at it. The mangy beast slunk away from him. A few moments later, I felt a tongue licking my ear. It then sort of climbed onto my shoulder, attached its front legs around my arm and started to do the things that dogs do, to my upper arm. It ruined the rhythm of my CPR. The dog seemed to be enjoying it but I most certainly was not! I heard the voice again. "Shurrup, gerorf, gerorf uv im."

And there I was, dressed for a promotion interview! We at last managed to get the patient breathing, the L/A clouted the dog, which reluctantly backed off me. With one eye on the dog in case it took a fancy to me again and hearing the chuckles of the L/A and doctor, we at last got the patient onto the stretcher and into the ambulance. The doctor thanked us for our help, or at least he started to thank us, but just then the dog started to sniff at his leg so he leapt into his car and left.

We at last delivered our patient to hospital and returned to HQ. I went to the gents and looked at myself. I stank of urine and dogs, my uniform was filthy, my shoes smudged with dog dirt. Just as I was about to attempt to get cleaned up, I heard a female voice shouting my name. I went out and met the girl who said they were ready for my interview. She pulled a face when she saw the state I was in. Looking little like a candidate for promotion, I walked into the office for the first of my many future promotion interviews.

I remember very little about that interview… but I did get the job!

CHAPTER TWENTY ONE

Pheasants

One of the advantages I discovered about living and working in the country, apart from the friendliness of the people, is to see, each day, the effect of the seasons on nature. I had no idea how little I knew about such things until I took up my new post.

As a 'towny' I had a completely unjust idea about country people, thinking them slow and dim-witted. I quickly found that I was very wrong when I moved to that small market town. I was now the Leading Ambulanceman and I had a chrome bar on each shoulder of my tunic to prove it. I was in charge of a station of two ambulances, three full-time (including me) and nine part time staff. I now looked at the post as an ideal stepping stone for further promotion, a good start for career development – I'd got the promotion bug! It didn't quite work-out as I had planned, because the town grew on me. I enjoyed living there and I spent far longer there than I had intended, but I enjoyed it, and that's what life's all about. My first sight of the station came as a bit of a shock... that is, when I actually managed to find the place. I had not expected it to be palatial, I'd not exactly come from an impressive establishment and was well aware that the County Council ran the Service on a tight budget, but it was still a shock. I had been up and down the road twice and eventually had to ask someone. If they hadn't pointed it out, I would never have guessed it was an ambulance station. I learnt that the building had started life as a slaughterhouse. During the war it had been taken over as an ARP post and at the end of hostilities it had been given to the Fire Service as a part-time station. They had moaned about its condition and two years prior to my arrival the building had been condemned when they built a new fire station. The old building had then been given to the Ambulance Service as a temporary residence. It was still temporary twelve years later when I left the County! I never dared ask where the ambulances had been kept before!

The station consisted of two garages, or more accurately two sheds, which took two ambulances. An ambulance could be backed into each with great care, but only close to the side wall, otherwise you could not open the door to get out. A small yard in front allowed us to wash down and park when not on the road. A desk at the back of one garage was to become my office. We had an arrangement with the pub on the corner to use their toilet. Of the two full time staff, Rob welcomed me at once with open arms. Rob, with his red face, deliberate and slow movements, was what I always thought of as a typical ambulanceman. Very mild tempered, he would go out of his way to help anyone and lend them his last shilling. He was great with kids and old people, in fact anyone needing attention; he fussed around the ladies and they all loved him. Rob was the sort of person you tell all your troubles to, what they call a good listener. He had married a local girl whom he had met when stationed near the town during the war.

When demobbed Rob had settled and taken a job in his old trade as a baker, joining the ambulance service about ten years before my arrival. Now and again he had a session in the kitchen and would delight in bringing something in for us. When he did this it was like birthday time as a kid.

"Just thought you might like a slice of chocolate cake for lunch mate," was Rob's favourite remark. A native of Wiltshire, his rolling accent betrayed his origin each time he spoke, a complete contrast to the local dialect.

Bert was a different type altogether. He was more than a little peeved that he'd not got the L/A's job, having expected it to be his as of right. Bert had also lost face with his mates, having told them he was to be in charge. The fact that 'his' promotion had gone to a man with less months service than Bert had years, had not gone down too well. But like most things, in time, Bert got over it. He had been brought up in a small village nearby and had started his working life as a Wagoner, in charge of the horses on a farm. It was his job to be up at dawn to feed them, look after them all day, and bed them down last thing at night. I suspect the war had come as the ideal opportunity to get away from the life and see the world, even if it was in the army. Bert had served his war in most campaigns. He and Rob would spend every opportunity yarning about differing parts of the world and the action they had seen, or arguing about the merits of their old infantry regiments. The fact that I had been a peacetime soldier, and a 'tanky' at that, meant I was out of the equation! Both men carried a proud array of ribbons on their uniforms. and although of different campaigns, each had the same number, I shudder to think what would have happened if one had had more than the other! Bert was all for getting the patients to their destinations and stopping for a pipe of 'baccy', whereas Rob refused to be rushed. The two would spend many an hour arguing the merits of how a particular patient should have been dealt with. Rob would delight in passing the time of day with everyone and was liked by all, Bert was inclined to be aggressive and brusque with people, that is until he met someone who he took to be an ex-army officer. He would then grovel and almost pull his forelock. On my second day I was summoned to go to the main station to meet my new boss, the Station Officer. He had been on leave when I was appointed so I had never met him, but I had heard a lot about him. Bert expounded long and hard about the man. I'd heard a great deal from all quarters and most of it appeared to be accurate.

    Quentin Farley could best be described as an exquisite man. He should have been an actor. He looked like one. Quentin was the epitome of a thespian, long wavy hair curling just above his collar, eyelashes the envy of every woman. Very slim, almost willowy, he was light on his feet and moved like a ballet dancer. When he walked, the top half of him seemed to stay still and his legs appeared to sway from the hips, and when he talked long slim hands and arms flowed as though he was conducting an orchestra. The station officer's shirts were sparkling white, always looking like an advert for a famous brand of washing powder, always with double cuffs and gold links bearing a coat of arms. Mr Farley's uniform was also exquisite, a perfect fit, an example of tailoring at it's best. I mentioned to him once that his was the only uniform in the Service that looked good. He winked and whispered "I know a clever little man in town". His voice, which was surprisingly bass and deep, was beautifully modulated, words flowing off his tongue, with a rolling of the r's. A simple utterance from Quentin was pronounced as though it was a delivery to the gods. His eyes were soft like a calf, but could blaze with an inward passion when roused. He was known as 'The Fairy Queen'.

I was to learn that Mr Farley's wife was even more attractive than he, the sort of woman you drive into lamp posts looking at. They had two small girls, each as pretty as their parents, each having the most perfect manners. They were a perfect and attractive family. Bert said Farley was as bent as a three speed walking stick, and I had to confess it was a little disconcerting at first, getting used to a man who called me darling, and to be told I was cheeky or naughty, but it was just Quentin's style. Mr Fairley never used bad language like everyone else, and to this day I am sure he was the most helpful and caring man I ever met. But I never understood how he became an ambulanceman. The Station Officer made me welcome and explained the running of the station. He made it abundantly clear that he would let me get on with my job and expected me to sort out routine problems, and not bother him.

"You've got a bar on your shoulder now dear, show me you know what to do with it!"

The first thing that struck me about living and working in a small town was how friendly people were. You said 'Good morning', and a few words as a matter of routine when you passed others in the street. You chatted about things when you went into a shop. I enjoyed going into a pub and finding I was made welcome. As it was only an hours drive away from my home I was able to travel daily until we found a house. We were lucky, our house sold quickly and I had only been working there about a month when I saw a bungalow that looked interesting. I arranged to take my wife over after tea and we both liked it at once, we knew it would suit us. Most unusually, we had no patients the next morning, so I was able to call into the Estate Agents and Solicitors to start things moving. Before I returned to the station, I called into the butchers for a pie for lunch. I then discovered what a small town was like when the lady assistant served me and said, "I hear you're moving into the Bell's bungalow" I was amazed!

We quickly settled into living in a small town and I found that ambulance work was a lot different in the country than in a town. In those days we never had designated emergency crews, we transported outpatients, and if an emergency came up, the nearest vehicle went. That meant we travelled a lot of miles each day. It took time to get to the scene and just as long to get the patient to the hospital. We had to be good to keep some patients alive.

The working pattern was to spend a week as a single crew on outpatients and two weeks as a double emergency crew. You still moved out patients but if you got a shout, you offloaded as soon as you could. Because of holidays and sickness, you were mostly part of the double crew. A few days alone as a single, was a luxury. The pace was slower, you had time to think, and you went in different directions and covered strange parts of the patch. Twice a week on the single vehicle, we had a regular afternoon run to a Rheumatic Clinic. This entailed a round trip of about a hundred miles, picking up patients from out of the way places, taking them to the Clinic for two o'clock and then waiting for them to have their treatment. It was a good chance to meet men from other stations, have a natter and compare notes. On the very odd occasion, you had to pair up and do a job. When that happened it meant a very late finish for no one else would take your patients home. When eventually everyone was ready you would start your return journey and take them home. The run started about midday and you got home about six, if all went well.

I very quickly got to know the patients on this run, they had all been going for years. The majority were middle aged to elderly ladies. Very few men attended for treatment, but I remember one old chap in particular.

Joe had been a farm labour all his life. Apart from a spell in the trenches during the First World War, he had never been out of the county. He spoke of the county town as I would speak of Australia. He was convinced that London was the haunt of 'criminals, gamblers and painted women'. I don't know how he imagined a 'painted woman', but he once whispered that one of my patients had been 'a bit of a lass as a young 'un'. Looking at the 80-year-old in question, her rosy red face under a woolly hat, dumpy shape and knobbly hands clasping the stout walking stick that gave her limited mobility, I found his words a little hard to believe.

Against all regulations, Joe always joined me in the cab. I enjoyed his company and was also very well aware his 'effing and blinding' did not go down too well with the ladies. No one could class Joe as a ladies man! My wife and I enjoyed our first meal of pheasant because of Joe. The farmers and gentry enjoyed a spot of shooting in that part of the world. I had always thought that shooting entailed a gun, a dog, muddy wellies and a lot of walking. I quickly learned that proper shooting is an industry. The birds are carefully raised and tendered from eggs. As they become of age they are encouraged to feed in certain areas. During the season a shoot would be organised with military precision, beaters would sweep the birds into the direction required where the 'guns' waited. It was a massacre, but it was part of country life and it gave employment to a lot of people. You bought a brace of birds from the game dealer, unless of course you had been a 'gun' yourself or knew someone. As ambulancemen, we still thought chicken was a treat.

"Pheasants are silly birds," Joe told me. He explained how easy it was to poach them, how, with a torch, to talk them down from trees at night as they roosted. He also told me how to make a simple trap with a bit of wire netting and string. The secret was a trail of corn and a low entry hole, the bird would always look up for escape, never down. I took his word for it but never tried! The first pheasant I enjoyed had been run over – well it would be more accurate to say it committed suicide. We were on our way back from the clinic run on a lovely fine evening in early spring. I'd had a job and we were running late, the old ladies had grumbled but the last had been dropped off and there was just Joe and I in the cab, enjoying a natter. A large grain truck had overtaken us and was in front. I expect the side wind from it disturbed the bird in the hedgerow, for the pheasant ran along the side of the truck flapping its wings as though trying to race the vehicle. Then, all at once, in a panic it took off and flew alongside the truck, and suddenly turned and flew straight into the side of it. The driver obviously never saw what happened and drove on. As soon as the bird bounced off the side of

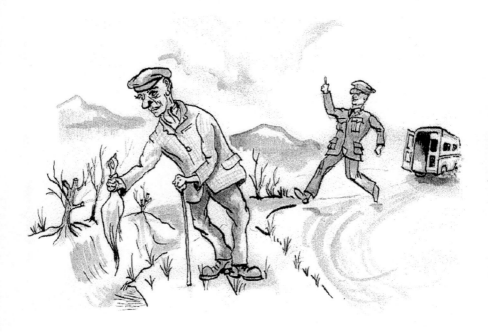

the truck and fluttered into the hedgerow, Joe started screaming for me to stop; he was already trying to get out before we pulled up! As soon as the wheels stopped he was off like a shot. For a man of almost eighty he could certainly move. He hobbled down the road as fast as his rheumaticy old legs and two sticks would take him. I let him beat me to it, I am sure I wouldn't have known what to do.

Joe reached the spot where the bird had bounced into the hedge and poked about with his sticks. It took him little time to find it. The bird had only been stunned and was fluttering feebly as he picked it up, with one quick move he snapped the bird's neck. He proudly held it up, a fine cock bird.

"There y'are boy, tek that ome t' missus."

So I did.

CHAPTER TWENTY TWO

The Maternity

I had now been at the little market town station for a number of months and was well into the working routine. The three of us worked Monday to Friday, 0830 until finished, six o'clock if you were on time, a lot later most days.

Nights and weekends were covered by 'stand-by'. This was a cheap method of obtaining cover in rural areas. A telephone was installed in your home and if an ambulance was needed Control rang you. You took the call, leapt out of bed and dressed quickly – you could always tell a standby crew as they wore black polo neck woollies in place of collar and tie – then a quick cycle ride to the station to collect the ambulance then off to do the job. After taking the ambulance back to station when finished, you returned to bed. It was not unknown to be out several times during one night. I can think of few things that are worse than just getting warm again, when the phone would ring! We were paid for this duty, and received the princely sum of five pence per hour on call and the hourly rate on a call out. They said it kept us fit, but 'they' were noticeably not the ones to be seen pedalling frantically through the frost in the early hours of the morning! Obviously three full time men could not cover every night and weekend, so we had auxiliaries – men who joined the Service as part of the standby rota after their normal working day. The nine auxiliaries at my station were an assorted bunch, good 'uns and bad 'uns. Like us, they had to hold a first aid certificate to prove they had been trained. On-station training was my responsibility as Leading Ambulanceman. The Fairy Queen came down about once a year to give them a pep talk, but in the main it was my job.

It was a little like the blind leading the blind and 'Dads Army' combined, but we did our best and as good a job as circumstances and resources allowed. It was my task to organise and try to make it as interesting as possible. Rob was always keen to help me, but Bert said it was not his job and kept well away. I tried hard to think up realistic exercises and hold discussion sessions about possible problems, but at times it was hard work. Every now and again someone would moan and point out that they did not get paid for training. I in turn learned my first lesson in management, and would explain that it was their responsibility to the town, and there were plenty of men to take their place if they wished to give up. As the job was held in high esteem amongst the local population no one ever took up my offer and left. Despite my new position of authority, knowledge gained through hands on experience, and the general broadening in my outlook, one thing bugged me.

Ask any ambulanceman how many road accidents he has attended, how many collapse cases he has been to, how many heart attacks he has dealt with? He will tell you he has no idea. But ask him how many babies he has delivered and he will tell you exactly! However, without being sexist, it doesn't have the same effect on the female staff as it does on the male. My first few months of inactivity did not last for ever. The very nature of the job quickly ensured that I attended, and dealt with, the whole range of accidents, injuries and misfortunes that happen to people. You name it, I and my colleagues dealt with it ... however one particular thing eluded me; whilst I had transported many, many maternity cases, I had never attended a birth or delivered a baby. Needless to say Ted, the man who had joined the same day as me, had dealt with dozens. Each time I went to a 'Matty' nothing happened. I got near to deliveries, but never near enough. The majority of my expectant mums would walk out to the ambulance and deliver the next day. On other occasions we would arrive at the house and a Doctor or Midwife would be there, having just delivered the baby. I could be paired up with a very experienced crew mate, the patient would be in advanced stages of labour, but still she would hold on until safely at the hospital. Twice within weeks I had finished a shift and the next crew would have a birth in the ambulance a few minutes after booking on duty. We could take a patient into a hospital who appeared to be well away from delivery, be having a cup of tea in the hospital kitchen and the nurse would breeze through and tell us it was a beautiful bouncing boy. But it never happened when I was there! It was almost as though it had been planned that I would never assist at a birth! Although I would never admit it to anyone I began to develop a fixation about childbirth. Why was it I was called to every type of incident apart from this particular one? I felt I was never going to see the miracle of birth. Needless to say, nowadays, ambulance trainees are instructed by Midwifes during training and attend hospitals to watch a delivery taking place, but this was not so in my day, the days of being trained were still far in the future. I had therefore been an ambulanceman for a good five years before it all happened, and I 'had a baby'.

It was in the early hours of a Monday morning when I received the call for the maternity. For some reason which I never quite understood, expectant mums always called us out in the early hours as opposed to during the day; someone said it was nature's way of getting back at the male sex who had caused the event! On this occasion, the patient was at another little market town nine miles away from us, the destination hospital twelve miles further. Control cheerfully said it sounded "very imminent" and we should "Get our skates on". My crew mate that night was an auxiliary called Bill. A nice young guy, he had only just started with us. Bill had taken the place of one of the stalwarts who had to retire. I had caused a lot of muttering when I insisted on advertising the post, holding interviews and selecting an applicant, being told in no uncertain terms that the next job always went to the next oldest member of the local voluntary aid unit. They were most put out that the new man was changing a system that had been working since the dark ages. I, however, dug my heels in and Quentin backed me. It was strange that the loudest voice for no change and to appoint as it had always been done, had come from Bert, but I reminded him that he had always said he would have 'Nowt' to do with the running of the station since I had beaten him to the job. Much to the horror of everyone, I appointed a young man to the post.

Bill was twenty one years of age, single, the owner of a most impressive sports car and had a succession of very attractive girlfriends. Each was a cracker but never lasted too long before being replaced by one with even better looks and longer legs. Obviously he knew all about babies at the point of conception, but undoubtedly far less than me at the delivery stage. As arranged I walked to my front gate and within a minute I heard the full throaty roar of the car as Bill screeched to a stop to pick me up. As usual he frightened the life out of me with the speed he took it through the deserted streets to the station. We left the station with the Bedford feeling noticeably sluggish after Bill's car, and made our way to our destination. After some searching we found the house tucked away in a narrow and dingy back street. We knocked at the door and walked in. As soon as I entered the small front room I knew my time had come. The good lady was on her hands and knees panting and moaning in front of the fire. I did not need the aged granny sitting in her rocking chair, nor indeed the College of Midwifes, had they been there, to tell me we were not going to make it this time. I rather optimistically asked if it was the first baby and groaned to myself when she panted. "No, the seventh" My time had come, a feeling of dread swept over me, I was not prepared for it. Although I had looked forward to the moment, I was not ready to deliver my first baby at that time of the morning, with a mate who had no idea at all! Nowadays they would have sent for the 'flying squad', but that name meant nothing to me at the time; such luxuries were yet to be invented. We very carefully loaded the patient onto our stretcher and into the ambulance. I did not need to tell Bill to request Control to inform the hospital and tell them what was happening, or to drive slowly and stop and join me when I called. With me looking far more confident than I felt, we set off on our long journey to the hospital.

The patient was very near to delivery, even I could tell that. I chatted to her attempting to reassure both her and I, whilst all the time fighting my panic and wishing I was (a) back in bed or (b) with a mate who knew what to do!

We had been taught to blanket the stretcher in a special way for a maternity patient. This enabled us to inspect the patient yet still leave the major part of her covered and warm. I found I was dreading what I would see if I looked under the blankets! At last, professionalism took over; I knew I had to do something, so taking a deep breath, I pulled down the blanket covering the lower part of her. The sight that appeared before my eyes is still with me today! I found myself staring at a thing like a wet, wizened, black walnut! It didn't look a bit like the 'crown' I had seen illustrated in my first aid books. Panic swept through me; this was the 'moment of truth'! I banged on the glass of the cab bulkhead and called to Bill to stop and join me, which he quickly did. I told him to open the 'maternity pack' I had placed on the bench by my side. Even today, every ambulance carries a 'Matpak', but in our day it was a brown paper parcel tied up with string! We were not allowed to open it unless a birth was imminent, but I had been told it contained all we needed. Unfortunately, it did not contain the most important ingredient... a midwife! Whilst Bill fumbled at his task of untying the string (I never understood why he didn't cut it) the baby was born. It chose the moment of birth with no help at all from me. It just came out! In fact it shot out – all I did was to catch it – a very small, very slippery, wet thing no bigger than my hands. One moment just a black scalp was showing, the next a baby boy was in my hands. I now understood the expression 'some women can give birth like shelling peas'. There was no question of holding baby up by its feet and smacking it as they did in films, this baby immediately demonstrated he had a powerful pair of lungs, opening his tiny mouth and announcing to the world he had arrived! I don't know who was the most surprised, the baby, his mother, me or Bill, who spun around at the sound. I am convinced, to this day, that he thought I had pulled it out quickly so that he missed seeing the birth!

I recovered from my shock and wrapped the tiny infant into an equally tiny blanket from the mat-pack. I passed it to Bill to hold, it was obvious he was not too sure about touching it. I then turned my attention to mum. She was fine. By the time you have produced as many babies as she had, I suppose you begin to get the hang of it. I gingerly touched the cord and gave a gentle tug. Nothing moved. Feeling that I had done enough for one night I decided to leave well alone and let the placenta stay where it was. Mum seemed happy and we were only ten minutes away from help. I made a snug little nest between mum's legs, and arranging the blankets to keep her warm and allow me to watch the baby, I told Bill to inform Control and continue. He did as he was told, but it was clear that he was in a sulk! I was fascinated, I'd never seen anything like this before. In those days, delivery was considered to be a female event, and fathers attending the birth of their children was unheard of. Mums went into the maternity home and you were left with instructions as to what time to telephone. The first I had seen of my own two sons, were as tightly wrapped blue bundles the following day in the arms of my wife. Until I became an ambulanceman I thought they came like that, scrubbed pink faces all screwed up and scowling, the wife saying "Isn't he gorgeous?" and me thinking 'no', but not daring to say so! This little bundle between his mother's legs was something very new to me. A round pink face, smeared with blood and mucus, the mouth open like a small bird, the raucous squawk demanding attention.

My earlier panic and lack of experience had now been forgotten. At long last I'd had 'my' baby and I was in charge of the situation again. I looked at the little face with an almost parental pleasure, immensely proud of the achievement, in fact in my mind it was developing into '*my* achievement'. I wiped a smear of blood from his cheek.

"Is he breathing alright?" asked mum.

I smiled and reassured her. By this time I was convinced there was nothing to it, it was all a mystique built up over the years.

"He's not deformed is he?" she asked.

I again assured mum that all was how it should be. I mused to myself, should I wake my wife when I got home and tell her how clever I had been. 'No,' I thought, perhaps she may not be that interested at this time of the morning.

"Is he all there? you know, as a boy, nothing's missing is it?"

I assured her he would be very proud of himself when he grew up. I then started to work out how I would slip it into the conversation at work that morning, or should I modestly say nothing and let them see the used matpak?

"You're sure he's breathing alright?" mother demanded. With the amount of noise the little fellow was making there was no chance of him not being all right. I again assured her all was in order. Trust your highly skilled ambulanceman, he's the expert. I touched the tiny chin and made clucking noises like you see women do when they see a new baby. It was then that the woman reduced my male ego down to the correct size and said.

"If he's alright, why are you staring at him so intently?" How could I, an ambulanceman, admit to my patient that it was because I'd never seen a new born baby before?

CHAPTER TWENTY THREE

The Wrong One

Idi Amin – we had never heard of him – the name sounded like something from a pantomime. We also had only the vaguest idea of where Uganda was, but one day we, together with the rest of the UK, woke up to find he was in all of the papers.

It was 1972, and in the matter of a few short days Idi Amin had expelled the Asian community from Uganda. The British government agreed to accept them, and in a very short time a very large number of confused and bewildered people were accommodated in disused military barracks. Within a radius of ten miles of our little town were many RAF stations, the county had been part of 'bomber country' during the war. The two nearest camps to our station were disused. They were on what the MOD called 'care and maintenance', which meant they were slowly falling apart. Within days these, and a number of others around the country, were hastily converted and full to overflowing with Ugandan Asians. Our workload went up many, many percent overnight, but of course, our resources remained the same, which warranted an explanation by management. Taff came over to the station one evening just as we were about to finish. He brought the Fairy Queen with him to explain what was required of us. He need not have bothered, it was simply summed up as 'extra work'!

The two men, in supposedly identical navy blue uniforms, could not have achieved a greater contrast. One immaculate, looking the part, unbelievably distinguished and elegant, the other looking as if someone had poured him into his uniform and missed! I escorted them to the corner of the garage that served as my 'office', pointedly ignoring the comment "Nice little place you got here boy-o," and offered them the two chairs, whilst I leaned against the bonnet of the ambulance. Rob brewed up before he went home, managing to find two reasonably clean and almost matching cups. Quentin pulled a face and looked as though he was worried about catching something, but Taff took his and drank without a second glance. The Chief explained the problem the Service now had and what was happening, which, it appeared, could be summed up as 'not a lot'. All the time Fairy Queen kept tut-tutting and murmuring.

"The poor dears, my heart bleeds for them. It must be so cold for them after being in a warm spot. I wonder if perhaps we could do a little knitting for them?"

We both ignored him. After I had been updated and had my moan, Taff beamed.

"Which is the best pub then kiddo... Fairy Queen's offered to buy us a beer!"

I was amazed the Chief referred to Quentin by his nickname, but he didn't seem to mind, only quickly adding, "I only mentioned a tiny half of bitter, dear,"

So we went to the Swan. I always drank in the Stomping Tomcat but I dared not take them there.

We had a good session, both men relaxed and talked non-stop. Taff had a fund of stories from when he was a scrum half, in a team Quentin had heard of but I, of course, hadn't. Taff had come from a village in the Rhondda and was proud of its good rugby club and choir. It also had 12 pubs and 8 chapels. He appeared to have belonged to them all, apart from seven of the chapels. It seemed his idea of a good Saturday was a game of rugby, getting knocked about followed by a night in the pubs. Sunday would be spent at chapel singing hymns, but he called them 'yims'. I recall his words, "We would yave a skinful after the game un roll yorm singing. My mum got very cross if we sang yims. She said yims wus for charpel and not for enjoyment!"

It was a pleasant session and the two proved to be good company. Although he didn't say a lot about his past I learned Quentin had achieved a good degree at Oxbridge. Following some time in the army he had been 'something in the City' but it had not suited him so he joined the Ambulance Service and moved to our County on promotion a little before the Chief. As they left he whispered to me, "Don't let that awful loud man Bert know I was an Army officer, it will ruin his image of me!"

The following day I told the others that the extra workload would have to be borne by us. If we couldn't take a joke etc... We collected our work details and headed for the ex-RAF station. We all felt very sorry for the Asians, as if being thrown out of their homes at short notice was not bad enough, coming from a hot country to the cold wilds of the UK and stuck in crumbling barrack blocks, disused for many years, must have seemed like the end of the world. Everyone tried their best to help and lessen the shock, but there was not a lot we could do. Workmen erected partitions, but there is little chance of making a barrack room seem homely, as any a squaddie will tell you. The voluntary aid societies, 'Sally Ann' and Social Services did their best, as did the NHS. Any large group of people will have health problems, these were no exception, and having left the heat of Africa for the UK did not help. Local medical resources were stretched to the limit and local ambulance crews were almost worn into the ground!

In addition to transporting people, we found we had the problem of finding them. As if that was not bad enough, few could speak English. We also discovered that even the most common names, similar to our Smith or Jones were completely unpronounceable. When you added to this problem the spelling of the name, usually guessed by the first person to write it down, and then changed many times as it was passed on from department to department prior to a transport request being made, mistakes could and did arise. At the sharp end the poor old ambulance crew, us, had no chance.

To add to the problem of names and the confusion surrounding them, people moved about within the barracks. It was perfectly understandable that people wished to be with friends and relatives instead of in the rooms to which they had been allocated, but nevertheless, this moving, combined with everything else, gave us problems we, nor the planners, had even dreamed of. Every day, we fought a losing battle with appointment times due to high demand and lack of resources, but the influx of Ugandans threw all attempts to keep to outpatient times out of the window. Each camp had a local person in charge, we never discovered their correct title, but always found a request for the 'Camp Commandant' produced someone to help us. I can well imagine that these hardy people would have been able to relate a number of interesting tales. When we received an emergency call at either site, the 'Camp Commandant' would always be on hand to take us to the patient, sort out the problems and explain to them they would be returned sometime. I only recall this system failing once.

We received a shout to a collapse one Saturday afternoon. This meant, of course, we were on standby at home. As my mate and I lived at opposite ends of the town, we had an agreement that the one farthest from the incident would collect the other. Grabbing tunic and cap, I leapt on my bike and pedalled furiously to the station to get the ambulance. With the engine screaming in protest, I swung the ambulance out of the garage and took off to collect Rob, who was waiting for me where his street met the main road. Switching on headlights, beacons and horns we took off for the camp. Imagine the scene... a warm Saturday afternoon and an RAF station in the middle of nowhere, the RAF always seemed to put their stations in the middle of nowhere, perhaps the airmen liked the peace and quiet. There was no place for the Asians to go, no transport, no telly, no nothing, the poor devils just sat about in the sun. So, when a shiny white ambulance swung into the gate looking like an illuminated bus on the seafront, it naturally caught their attention and they came to see what was happening. Our vehicle was quickly surrounded by a sea of black faces, each chattering twenty to the dozen to each other and to us, not an English voice or face to be seen. Of course we had no address other than the camp and the message said we would be directed to the patient.

Our plea for someone who could speak English made no sense to them, all we got was a babble of voices and waving arms. Just as Rob was about to call for help on the radio, a tall and distinguished gentleman dressed in what had been a smart suit, pushed his way to the front. In an accent reminiscent of Peter Sellers, he said, "Pleased to be of following me kind sirs." I thanked him and asked what was wrong with the patient. He told me she was very, very ill and may perhaps be dying. Our guide pointed to a barrack block on the far side of the square and proceeded to push his way through the throng. We followed as quickly as the crowd would allow, which was pretty slow. At last we stopped outside the block and struggled out of the cab. Collecting our small carry chair and a blanket we followed him into the block. Maybe it was not quite accurate to say we followed, for the crowd almost carried us into the building, into the foyer, up the stairs and down a corridor until we reached the room. With a bow, the tall gentleman ushered us in. It had been an NCO's room, designed for one person. Inside were two single beds, an old man, a young woman and at least a dozen kids of assorted shapes and sizes, and on one of the beds lay an old lady. I'd never before thought of a dark person looking pale, but she did, she was obviously very ill.

We managed to shoo the other people out of the room apart from our guide and examined the patient. Rob requested oxygen. I had to force my way through the crowd to the ambulance to get the portable set and then back to the room. As I re-entered the room the crowd tried to came in with me. It took a lot of pushing and shouting to clear them out to allow us to work on the patient. We gave the patient oxygen and after a few minutes, she seemed in a better condition and fit to move. Placing the blanket onto the chair we lifted her off the bed onto the chair and tucked her in. She was a light as a feather. It was time to leave. Our escort opened the door, and with that everyone surged into the room! With more shouting and waving of arms our escort found room for us to move. I am convinced that our feet never touched the ground. The mass of the crowd seemed to carry us along the corridor, down the stairs and into the ambulance. It took some minutes to make every one understand that we needed room to transfer the patient onto the cot. At long last we succeeded, made her comfortable and prepared to leave for the Hospital. As the lady could speak no English we were happy to take our escort but refused to take the two dozen relatives and friends who wanted to break the afternoon with a ride out. It was in the midst of this long and loud debate that we suddenly spotted a white face and above the babble of voices heard an authoritative voice booming out above the noise.

The lady in question had the style and charisma of one used to dealing with lesser mortals and gaining immediate obedience. The people parted before her like waves before an approaching battleship. The words of a song made famous by Joyce Grenfell flashed into my mind, 'Stately as a galleon'. Her forceful bosom gave her a presence that no lesser mortal would dare to argue with. Her eyes took in the scene and rested on me.

"What..." she boomed "...are you doing?"

Whilst it seemed a pretty silly question, the situation became one of officer and other rank, with me very much the junior. I explained we were taking the patient into A&E. The patient had by now disappeared under the blanket. The voice boomed again.

"It was I who called you. I have been waiting for you by the patient's bedside. You have the wrong person."

I looked at our erstwhile guide who was now bowed with his hands held before him as though in prayer.

"Memsahib, my mother wishes to go to the hospital," he said.

The man seemed to shrivel before the gaze of the mighty one. The silence could have been cut with a knife, after a moment our erstwhile guide spoke rapidly in a strange tongue to the inert form on the cot. To our amazement the old lady, who had been at death's door a few moments ago, threw back the blankets and climbing off the cot scurried away, seemingly as fit as I was!

By now the crowd had pulled back to a respectful distance, and our guide now vanished. The lady escorted us to another barrack block. As she advanced, with us following in her wake, the crowd fell respectfully away from her. She took us into another block where we collected our collapse case. We didn't dare say it, but the young lady who walked out looked far fitter than the last person who had occupied the cot!

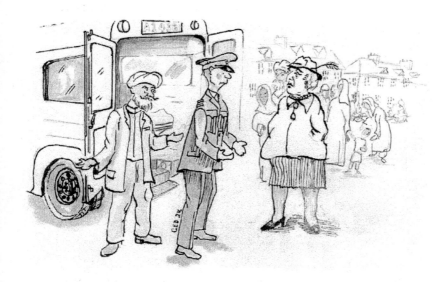

CHAPTER TWENTY FOUR

Pheasants II

You could tell the season of the year from the type of vegetables we ate, often with great regularity, the kids complaining about getting them so often acting as a reminder.

Ambulancemen were never given tips of cash, apart from the odd half-crowns the old people would give us. These were always the people who could least afford it but they became most upset if you refused. I was shown that it was easier to accept and then slip the coin under a cushion or newspaper for them to come across later. In that way, no one lost face and we did not feel guilty. We did, however, receive vegetables and fruit, lots and lots of them. Everyone living in the countryside seemed to grow vegetables, and they were not at all like the tasteless things you buy nowadays in the supermarkets. Not only did our regulars give us samples of their produce, they seemed to be under the impression that we were gourmet diners, questioning us on the finer points of taste and texture when we next collected them. As I said, we used to work one week alone, and two as the emergency crew. The single week was the one where we transported outpatients, mainly elderly people, and these were the ones who gave us the fruits of their labours. It was not at all uncommon for the 'sitting bus', as we called it, to return in the evening looking like the back of a mobile shop. The spoils were then shared out to the tune of, "Bert, Mrs Cross said she wants to know if these beans are as good as last year." and "Rob, I've got strict instructions to tell you to try these apples, Mr Wilson said they are far better than the things old Mrs Jones gave you last week, and if you think they are nice would your good lady like some more and make him a pie?"

The conversations ran like that most of the time. We were well aware that these gifts were the patients way of thanking us for our help. The vast majority had very little money but they knew how to live off their gardens, and would have been offended had we refused what they offered us. A number were very good poachers too, and it was not unknown for us to take a brace of rabbits or a pheasant home. We, in turn, did our best to help people find their way around the hospital departments and clinics, and sort out their next appointments. We would fetch prescriptions and check their appliances were in order before we took them home. When we collected and returned patients, it was all part of the job to turn the gas off and light it on their return, put the cat in or out, put the kettle on the gas or bring in a bucket of coal. We were also well known at a number of village post offices and shops where we stopped to collect pensions or bread and milk. All the time I spent at that country station I never managed to get over how grateful people could be to us for just helping them a little. I was also very aware that a number of old people saw no one from when the ambulance left their home until it called for them again. It was all part of the job of being an ambulanceman.

It was the late afternoon of a beautiful day as Rob and I returned to town after an uneventful day as the emergency crew. Whilst there was still plenty of time left for us to get a job, we were both looking forward to an evening off. Rob was a keen gardener and I always found something to do around the house. As we approached the main crossroads we saw the sitting bus approaching from the other direction. We flashed our lights to give him right of way. As he turned into the road in front of us to the station Bert waved excitedly to us, his round face slit from ear to ear with a big beam. He was obviously bursting to tell us something, or had possibly been given a load of produce to share out. We slowed down to allow him to swing into the station yard first and reverse to the garage door and then followed him in. Before we could get out of the cab Bert was at the driver's window, full of himself.

"I was coming down Thorpe Lane by Fox Covert when these two cock pheasants took off, I tell you, they were like two Spitfires. They swooped low over Crowson's greenhouse, swung round that great oak and came straight at me".

Rob grinned, "I hope you made sure there were no police cars around mate."

He was referring to an incident before my time that Bert had never been allowed to forget. It seemed he was on his own on the back roads and there, miles from anywhere, he came across a magnificent cock pheasant dead in the middle of the road. Bert hit his brakes and as he did glanced into his rear view mirror. He was annoyed to see a police car following in the distance. Now we had a good relationship with the law, but Bert was of the old school: 'never trust a copper'. He took his foot off the brake and proceeded to drive slowly along the road. In due course the patrol car passed him and the driver pipped its horn. As soon as the car was out of sight Bert turned in a farm gate and drove quickly back to claim his prize, but of course it had gone. Bert never forgave that copper!

Bert was not going to have his tale interrupted, and pointedly ignored Rob's words. His eyes shone with excitement, he was enjoying the attention of being centre stage. With both arms outstretched, his body swung like an aircraft as he demonstrated the bird's flight.

"Damn things came straight at me. I thought they wus going to come straight in through the dang 'screen. I braked, but you know how narrow yon lane is there, 'tween the 'edges. Them dang birds must have been intent on committing suicide. Last second they swung low. Wallop! they clouted the bumper and shot either side of the bus".

"Did it mark the paint" I asked, ever mindful of the paperwork an accident entailed.

"Sod the paint, its nowt. I wus out like a shot, got 'em both, smashing birds all ready for the pot, come and have a look"

Bert proudly swaggered around to the back of the ambulance with us following. Always one for dramatics, Bert paused a smirk on his face, then with a flourish like a conjurer producing a rabbit from a hat, he swung open the back door to show off his prizes. We scattered as, with wings clattering, two alarmed cock pheasants took flight between us, squawking and shrieking, and we watched as Bert's supper took off over the station roof, scared but otherwise none the worse for their ride in a County Ambulance. The two birds had obviously only been stunned, and Bert in his excitement had not checked to see if they were dead.

Needless to say, the inside of the ambulance was full of feathers and bird droppings as the two had regained consciousness and attempted to escape. Bert's language was unprintable and Rob's comment "Should you report it to the police?" did not go down well with him either.

Of course, we were never to let Bert live this incident down.

CHAPTER TWENTY FIVE

The Bill

With a gleam in his eye and an exaggerated flourish, Bert threw the official looking envelope down on to my desk.

"If I'm gonna 'ave to pay to come to work, I wanna pay rise!"

At the best of times he was a great one for talking in riddles, but now Bert had our attention he was going to make the most of it. I looked inside the buff-coloured envelope and his words fell into place as I read the enclosed form.

It all started on a beautiful summer's evening, the sort that makes you feel you ought to be 'doing something in the garden'. I had finished the day's work and, as was often the case, was on stand-by at home. Having had tea, I was walking the petrol-driven lawn mower up and down the piece of field that was called my back garden. I was not at all interested in gardening and would never in my wildest dreams have called the expanse of rough grass a lawn. The term lawnmower was also rather a misnomer. It was not old enough to be an antique, it could not even be called second-hand, for it had been in Rob's possession for years, and he could not even recall how he got the thing. Rob had mentioned that he had been going to throw it away so I begged it from him. Another mate who liked to tinker with things, had played with the workings of the machine for ages and made it work... well more or less work. To say it had long since seen better days was being polite. I hated the effort of cutting the grass, and apart from that, I would spend longer pulling and recoiling the cord to start the ancient two-stroke motor than I would cutting the grass. I was not at all pleased when my eldest son started to run alongside, waving his arms, trying to attract attention. I would have to stop the machine to hear what he wanted and I knew that it would be a swine to re-start if I did. Only when he mimed putting his hand to his ear did I realise he was trying to tell me that the telephone was ringing. I pushed the switch on the machine to stop and left it coughing and spluttering as I ran into the house. Needless to say, it was Control... they had found an RTA for me.

I took the details from Control and, following the usual system, asked them to tell Bert I would wait for him at the roadside as usual. As he would be picking me up, I had time to wash my hands and make myself a little more presentable. I reached the corner and realised it was a very still summer's evening now that my mower had finally stopped! I waited for a couple of minutes, leaning against a tree and thinking about nothing, before I heard the ambulance approaching. As I climbed in, Bert switched on lights and beacon and put his foot down. We had just taken delivery of a brand new Ford Transit Ambulance and were still enjoying the refreshing turn of speed it gave after our old 'bus'. The RTA was about ten miles away down very twisting lanes. Bert took them with skill and care. He had worked the patch for years and knew every inch of road;

he knew where he could cut corners by using peripheral vision, and where the bad bits were. We had the approximate location of the RTA and a good idea of where it would be. It never ceased to amaze me how people would miss the same bend or go into the same stretch of dyke; we could generally pinpoint the spot where an accident was likely to be, and were not often wrong. A fresh gap in the hedge and two parked cars had me reaching for the radio to inform Control we had arrived at the scene, and once again, it was where we had guessed it would be. I grabbed my box and jumped out, slithering down the grassy bank towards the car that had managed to wrap itself around the only tree in the field. An elderly couple stood nearby and a young man was kneeling by the driver's door. They all started to tell me what had happened.

With half an ear listening to them, I made a quick reconnoitre of the scene and injuries. The driver was unconscious and obviously trapped by his feet in the wreckage. His female passenger was having hysterics. She was making so much noise she could not have been too badly injured. You quickly learn that it is the silent ones you have to concentrate on; if someone has the strength to make a lot of noise, it is a fair bet they are not too badly injured. I told the young man to get back to Bert and ask him to request the Fire Brigade and to bring me the resuscitator, the patient's respiration being poor. Bert quickly joined me and passed the good news that not only was a fire crew on the way but Gordon, a local doctor and a good friend of ours, one who always liked to help, had been alerted and was well on the way. The condition of the trapped patient was deteriorating and Gordon would be invaluable. Those were days long before anyone had thought of paramedics. By the time we had got an airway into the patient and checked out his injuries Gordon had arrived. A big advantage of working in a country patch rather than a town, was that we all knew each other, having worked together a number of times, and we all knew each other's capabilities. In a very short time, Gordon had established a saline drip and it was reassuring to see it start to have an effect.

At this point we heard the sound of horns and knew the fire crew had arrived.

I always had the greatest admiration for the way those lads could cut a car apart and release a patient for us. We quickly liased and they started on the complicated task of getting the driver out. We had worked with the crew before, but on this occasion, I detected a number of worried looks pass between them. Bert had taken the female patient to the ambulance and the doctor was bent over the patient listening to his chest. I was wedged in the car at the back of the patient holding a drip with one hand and the oxygen mask over the patient's mouth and nose with the other, a position where I could watch his condition and ensure it did not worsen.

I noticed a fireman standing by my side, apparently doing nothing, and took no notice of him – it meant nothing to me that he was holding a fire extinguisher. I then realised another fireman was wrapping a heavy fireproof sheet around me. I'd been on the job long enough to know they that don't mess about, and looked askance at him. The Sub-Officer in charge leaned close to me and whispered into my ear.

"Just a minor precaution mate, the battery's between the engine block and the tree, we can't isolate it. A fuel line is leaking petrol onto the patient's feet, and when we make the final snip, there could be a spark. Don't worry though I've got a guy with an extinguisher and if anything happens we'll get you out!"

Under the circumstances, I thought it was a pretty silly thing to say don't worry! Suddenly the birds seemed to stop singing and I'm sure it turned colder. The Sub whispered to Gordon who, giving me a sheepish grin, stepped back.

"They know what they're doing mate, I'll be here."

So there I was, wrapped up like a mummy inside a car which might perhaps be about to burst into flames, holding a patient who was, fortunately, not aware of what was happening, and everyone was stepping back telling me not to worry! I looked down at the fireman kneeling at the patient's feet with what looked like an extra large pair of pliers. I prided myself on being cool in emergencies, that was my job, but there are emergencies and emergencies. Had my time come at last?

"Ready?" the fireman asked.

I wasn't, but said "Yes."

With a deep breath he clipped the final bit. I held my breath for what seemed to be half an hour.

Nothing happened, and I started to breathe again. It took little time for them to release me and for us to ease the patient free and load him onto the stretcher. Many willing hands carried it up the bank to the ambulance. Bert had got the female settled down by then, but as soon as she saw the man she started to panic again. Gordon stabilised the patient in the back of the ambulance and gave something to the woman which quietened her down a little and at last we were able to leave the scene for the hospital.

The accident had been on the farthest corner of our patch, as a result the nearest hospital we could take them to was one we used very infrequently. We knew where it was and how to find A&E but that was about all. Whilst I worked on the two patients, Bert informed Control and requested the hospital be notified of the patient's condition and our arrival time. They were waiting for us as we drew in, and helped us to unload. As usual, the system worked, and within minutes our male patient was wheeled into a theatre and the female into a cubicle. Bert and I started the routine of sorting out the back of the vehicle ready for the next job, sweeping out the mass of grass and mud we had managed to collect and replenishing our kit. The back of an ambulance after an emergency always looked a mess. Working in the country, we seemed to have picked up an acre of hayfield as well and it looked worse than usual, but we were used to this and very quickly had all in order. Dirty and bloodstained washing was placed into a pillow case and pushed under the stretcher for soaking in water when we got back to the station before sending to the laundry. Clean blankets were dragged out of lockers and made ready. In no time, we were organised and ready for our next job… so off we went in search of tea.

We found an obliging nurse who took pity on us, had just telephoned Control and each had a mug of steaming tea in our hands when a lady in a white coat found us. Were we the crew who had brought in the RTA? When we confirmed we were, she asked who was the driver and I pointed to Bert. We were both a little surprised when she asked for his name and address. Bert gave it to her, and just as he was about to ask why, a porter called to say Control had telephoned and we had an urgent admission. We left in a hurry.

Bert wondered why his name had been taken, but we assumed it was some sort of routine at that particular hospital, perhaps they were going to send a Christmas card! We both forgot all about it as job followed job and we fretted about getting home.

Three weeks later Bert received a bill from the hospital for emergency medical treatment, and slapped it on my desk!

It is standard NHS procedure to send an account for emergency medical treatment to drivers involved in an RTA. This amount is determined by the Department of Health and the cash goes to the receiving hospital. The number of people who think it is for the ambulance never ceases to amaze me. It is a pity it isn't, for it would have funded a lot of things we needed and never got. The cash is claimed from the car insurance as a matter of routine, but it is a procedure that gives a lot of people the impression that they are having to pay for the ambulance.

It would appear that on the evening we took our RTA to the hospital, a new receptionist had started her first evening in the reception department. As she had been left on her own, it had been impressed upon her that if an RTA came in she must get the name and address of the driver. No one had said which driver!

CHAPTER TWENTY SIX

Brazil Nuts

They say it takes all sorts to make the world go round. In Yorkshire they also have a very true saying: 'Tha's nowt as queer as folk'. There is nothing like the back of an ambulance to prove the truth of these statements.

Our morning run every day contained a number of day-hospital patients, elderly people who spent the day at a special unit where they were looked after. They received medical attention, had a hot bath, hot meals and an opportunity to talk to other people. We collected them mid-afternoon and returned them to their own home by teatime. It was a change of scene to the old folk, and gave a break to those looking after them. It was a sad fact of life that some people we took a liking to whereas others could be a 'pain in the neck'. Our job was to transport them and whether we liked them or not, we did our best to look after them. One morning a new name appeared on our list. Mr Padfield lived in a ramshackle cottage miles from anywhere. We prided ourselves on knowing our way around our 'patch', but even so, his home took a bit of finding. A green lane off a desolate country road slowly turned into a dirt track between flat fields. After a mile this ended in what appeared to be a disused farmyard, with old barns and buildings in assorted stages of collapse and rusted cars and farm machinery that would have been eagerly accepted by any rural museum, had they but known where to find them. If it had not been for a scruffy mongrel dog barking at the end of a length of chain fixed to the old oil barrel which served as it's kennel, we would have thought the place was deserted.

The thought of fighting our way to and from this place every day, especially with winter coming on, was not one we wished to dwell upon. We climbed out of the cab into a soft glutinous mud, which threatened to cover our shoes, and paddled to the house. I banged on the back door and was not surprised to receive no response. Not knowing what to expect, we pushed open the door and shouted "Ambulance!"

A croak from the depths of the house told us he was at home. Unfortunately, like the homes of so many old people, the place was a tip. On every flat surface, dirty pots and pans, piles of old newspapers, tins and packets of food fought for the available space or lay on the floor where they had fallen. Furniture fit only for the rubbish dump was crowded into every part of the room, competing with old bikes and bits of farm machinery. The building had that unique smell of very old and neglected country cottages, damp, cold, paraffin, tobacco and rancid fat. Sat in a big old Windsor chair by the meagre fire, surrounded by old newspapers and dirty cups and plates, was a scrawny and grubby old man. His face was gaunt and pinched, his beak-like nose gave him the resemblance of a bird of prey.

Mr Padfield was dressed in assorted layers of shirts, pullovers, waistcoats and shawls. Greasy trousers almost reached the tops of his large working boots and a fat ginger cat, far better fed than he, sat on his bony knees, scowling at us as if defying us to enter.

It was obvious that the old man lived alone in this one downstairs room. The inner room was half a degree warmer, mainly because it was crammed full of furniture. In the centre was a large double bed, piled high with soiled bedding and clothes. Next to it was an equally large table covered in a dark blue chenille table cloth. Unlike the clutter of the rest of the rooms, it was empty, except that, in the centre, rather incongruously, stood a large cut glass bowl. Having ascertained we had found the right patient, we helped Mr Padfield into a voluminous and very ragged ex-army greatcoat, wrapped his muffler around his neck, (old men always had mufflers rather than scarves), and put a greasy cap on his head. We found his glasses, put them on his nose and slowly helped him out to the ambulance. Mr Padfield became one of our regulars. As the weeks went by we got to know him very well. When he was the last patient to take home, I would love to sit in the back with the old boy and listen to his tales of life in the trenches during the First World War. Like most of his generation, he had left the farm to do his bit in the war, eager to see "a bit o 'em furiners afore it ended at Christmas." Four years later, after serving in the thick of the bloodiest battles, Henry Padfield was one of the lucky ones who returned home. In time he had married a local girl and they had set up home in this cottage miles from anywhere. From then on, they never went further than the local market town once a week.

We learnt our patient had retired and since his wife had died many years ago, lived alone with Percy the cat. A neighbour brought his shopping in and visited him twice a week. Apart from that, us, and the day hospital, Percy was his only contact and obviously received more attention than his owner. As the years passed and age had taken its toll he had retreated into the one room, and lived with his memories. The cut glass bowl had been his wife's pride and joy. Despite the clutter all over the room, the bowl was the only thing allowed on the table, it was almost like a shrine dedicated to her. We noticed one day the bowl contained an amount of shelled and broken Brazil nuts. As he got to know us, he would offer them to us. Bert and I always declined for we hated nuts, but Rob loved nuts. Every time we collected Mr Padfield, or took him home, he would offer us some. Rob always took a handful.

It was one bitterly cold morning with sleet in the air and a cold wind sweeping across the fields that Rob, nibbling nuts, chanced to remark as we walked him slowly out of the house.

"You like your Brazil nuts Mr Padfield."

The old man stopped and looked at him.

"No I don't!" he said.

We took a few more paces to the ambulance.

"But you must" insisted Rob. We stopped again, the wind pulling at our coattails and caps.

"Why must ah?" Henry Padfield demanded.

"Cos you always have a bowl full," Rob said, with a smile.

It was obvious to me that the old man was getting cross.

"Shut up Rob," I hissed, but Rob, happily chewing nuts, was not to be silenced and continued.

"But, you must like 'em Mr Padfield. You always have the big bowl full, and I only wondered why you kept buying them if you don't like them." Rob insisted.

"I don't buys em," the old man said, "Fred my neighbour gets 'em fer me."

I was more than ready to accept his word, knowing how old people have strange ways and fixations, but Rob would not let it drop.

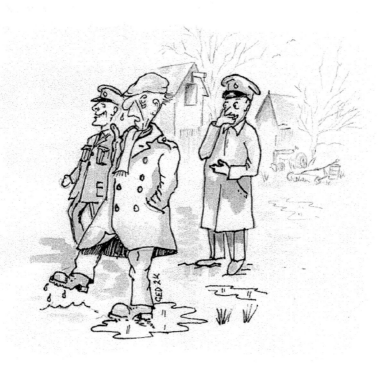

"But Mr Padfield, if you don't like them, why don't you tell your neighbour not to get you any more of them?"

We stopped again. I was losing my patience with the pair of them. We were late, we had a number of people yet to collect, and it was cold stood in the farmyard. The old man looked up at Rob with pity in his watery old eyes, a drew drop shimmering on the end of his hawk like nose. He spoke slowly, as though talking to a backward child.

"I tells yer, I don't like em, old Fred knows I don't like em, but he knows I do like toffee."

By then both Rob and I were lost. Mr Padfield paused whilst we all struggled to keep upright as a gust of wind unhindered in its travel across the North Sea, tried to take us into the middle of the yard. As the wind abated a little he spoke again.

"I knows yer likes Brazil nuts, cos yer told me, so I tells Fred ter get Brazil nut toffee. I don't like the darn things, but I don't spit 'em onter the fire no more, I spits 'em into the Missus' bowl and saves em for you!"

I'll never forget the look on Rob's face, it was a picture. I never saw him eat another nut after that day!

CHAPTER TWENTY SEVEN

China Tea

As I have already mentioned, the main aim of all ambulance staff is to drink the maximum amount of tea. Crews quickly learn never to refuse a cuppa, you never know when you'll get a chance for another one!

It was a beautiful Monday morning in early June. The weather was perfect and still, and everything looked good. It made you feel glad to be alive, and to think about holidays rather than work. We had only had one discharge to clear from the hospital that morning, which was most unusual for a Monday. We had taken a steady ride into the City, met our patient on the ward and taken him home. He had proved to be a most interesting old chap and I had enjoyed our chat on the journey. Leaving him safe and sound, we made our way back to the station. It looked like being one of those rare occasions when we could catch up with a few chores when we got back. We cruised along in no hurry, with the cab windows open, enjoying the pleasure of country lanes, lack of traffic and the sights and sounds of country life. It was an attractive part of the county, and on Sundays it would be packed with cars as everyone escaped into the country. On working days such as that Monday, the roads were empty.

We were not surprised when the radio came to life to spoil things. Control called with a priority, an RTA with a reportedly trapped patient, police and fire crew already en route. We were used to such events and speedily headed in the required direction. It was not too far away which was fortunate. Rob put his foot down, but knowing the patch well, we were well aware that excess speed and emergency horns were out of the question on these roads.

Within minutes we turned the corner and saw the accident. By the side of a picturesque cottage (the sort you only see in books nowadays) a car had missed the sharp bend to finish with its bonnet deep into a dyke. Two old ladies dressed in tweeds and cardigans, looking as though they had stepped from the pages of *Country Life* magazine, stood by the car, frantically waving for us to slow down. As we pulled up, a police car approached from the other direction, which further delighted and excited the old ladies. Whilst Rob positioned the ambulance, I took my box and went to the side of the car. One old lady said the girl in the car seemed alright but she could not get out. Her companion proudly declared she had driven an ambulance during the war and should she put the kettle on? Always keen to get rid of bystanders, I agreed that it would be a lovely idea. The pair left just as the policeman joined me. He nodded, said "Ow do," and together we slithered down the grass to the side of the car, which was a large and very expensive sports saloon. I heard the copper mutter, "What a motor! Fancy putting a thing like this in a dyke."

The driver's window was open and as we edged to it we saw the driver, an extremely attractive and very worried-looking girl of about twenty, looking anxiously at us from behind the steering wheel. It was very apparent to me, and she also assured me it was so, that she was unhurt, but she could not get out of the car. It was stuck with both doors firmly wedged against the sides of the dyke. The young lady was most concerned about causing trouble to us and seemed embarrassed to have warranted an ambulance and a police car. The copper muttered, "Wait until she sees the fire crew!"

The poor girl explained that, swerving to miss a pheasant, she had gone straight into the dyke. She was shaken and understandably worried about what her father would say about his new and very expensive car. Through the window, I checked to ensure she was not injured in any way and had not previously been unconscious. It was going to be an expensive insurance job, but as no one was hurt we were happy.

Scrambling back to the ambulance I radioed Control and suggested we stand by, for getting the car out of its resting place could involve some risk to the rescuers. They okayed it, telling us to keep a listening watch in case needed. With that the Fire Appliance turned up with, naturally, a full crew. Almost at the same time a tractor drove along the lane and pulled up to see what all the excitement was about. While all of this was going on, the two old ladies peered excitedly at us through their window. The fire officer liased with the policeman and I, and it was decided that, as the girl was trapped, we could not risk waiting for a breakdown truck. They would attach a length of chain to the back axle of the car, the other to the tractor and drag it out of its resting place. Positioning myself on the bank side to be near the girl, and well out of the line the car would move, I waited for the fire crew and farmer to start the exercise. It was a long time since I had sat on the grass in the sun chatting to a pretty girl – it was just a shame about the circumstances!

As always at an incident, everyone worked together and improvised, the tractor had come along at a very fortunate time. At last, with firemen at strategic points, the operation started. It all worked very well and the car was dragged out with no mishaps to anyone or anything apart from the paintwork. 'Daddy' was not going to be pleased!

In no time the shaking girl was helped from the car. We double-checked she was not harmed, and I was not surprised when she declined to go to hospital for a check-up. At that point our elderly ladies reappeared and announced the kettle had boiled and would we like to go into the cottage for tea. The fire crew, in full fire fighting kit, were reluctant but were persuaded by the ladies, who were clearly enjoying the excitement. Escorting our patient, Rob and I led the procession up the garden path and into the cottage. The cottage was of the sort you see on postcards: all chintz, expensive carpets and antique furniture. Into this attractive but tiny room crowded the patient, two ambulancemen, two policemen, five firemen, a farmer and the two lady owners. The older of the two ladies sat the girl down, placed a cup and saucer in her hand and asked, "China or Indian?"

The girl politely said "China," and a teapot looking like something from a museum was instantly produced. The other lady asked me the same question and I had no idea.

Although we drank endless cups of tea, my education as to where it came from was sadly lacking, although I did wonder if Typhoo was a country. The girl had said China, so I too said. "China, please."

Rob quickly followed my lead, followed by every one else. It was obvious that no one wanted to show themselves up! The old ladies seemed delighted and rushed about with teapots. A moment later I was given a tiny and fragile cup and saucer and was horrified to see a thin green liquid carefully poured in. I was not alone, the faces of my colleagues in the other Services showed they too were more than a little surprised! I looked around, but seeing neither sugar nor milk, said nothing and drank as if it was my normal tipple. It tasted foul. I noticed the others looking around, following suit and pulling faces. In this crowded room, among the large group of uniformed, uncomfortable and sweating men, the two old ladies twittered between us, passing small plates, small cakes and pouring fresh cups of the strange and horrible green stuff. It must have been the most exciting day those old ladies had experienced for many years. As they passed, I overheard one whisper to the other, "I never realised how knowledgeable these men are about tea."

How little did she know!

CHAPTER TWENTY EIGHT

Bathrooms

We seemed to spend a lot of our time in the bathroom. It was amazing the number of jobs we got that involved bathrooms. I often wondered what people did in there, apart from the obvious. I was quite convinced, at times, that if people felt ill they would drive home and go into their bathroom before they collapsed and waited for someone to send for us. Very often they seemed to get wedged behind the door, just to give us something else to do.

One of the characteristics of the British is their insistence on privacy, and I confess to being one of them. Experience has taught me that when the majority of people go up to the bathroom for a bit of privacy, they can be gone for hours before anyone thinks to check if they are OK, and then of course they find the door has been locked. The number of jobs we had in these situations borders on the unbelievable.

One of the problems with most bathrooms is size. Large bathrooms are very few and far between, and to make matters worse, the door always opens inwards. May I suggest that the next time you are in yours, having a quiet think, study how much floor space you have, and then imagine how someone could get the door open if you were laid out in that space.

Everyone has heard the tale of the glamorous blonde with her toe stuck in the water tap, so have I, but I regret to say I never dealt with her; shame about that! But we did once have a job with a lady stuck in the bath. This good lady was a little overweight, in fact more than a little, she was about five feet tall and eighteen stone. One day she got stuck in the bath. It appears that due to her size it was a great struggle for her to get in and out of the bath so she would not lock the door and her husband would help when required. They were like a married couple in one of those old-fashioned seaside postcards, a very fat lady and a skinny little man. On the evening in question, the lady had decided to have her bath and had been helped in by hubby. When she had finished she called him and he attempted, without success, to get her out. She was well and truly stuck, she was so big that her large amounts of fat had become wedged in the bath. In addition, the water had become trapped beneath her and causing a suction action. It was not at all funny for the poor lady and most embarrassing. How long she was stuck there before they plucked up courage to get help, I never knew, but at last they decided to call for assistance. However, the question arose, who to call? At last hubby decided that the fire service was their best choice. She did not agree, for as it was a small market town, the fire service was a retained crew, all local people, and they would know her. She just could not face the embarrassment. Having decided that the ambulance service would be safer, he dialled 999 and said it was a collapse.

I was on call with old 'arry, we met at the station and went to the scene. Harry of course knew everyone, and consequently knew the lady in question. We were let in the front door, and the husband explained his wife's predicament as we went up stairs to the bathroom. I had to smother a grin when hearing the details of the situation, but as soon as I saw the lady I realised it was not at all funny. The water was going cold and the patient was in danger of suffering hypothermia. I sent 'arry for a blanket and we tucked this around her. This gave us a little leverage but not enough for us to extricate her from the bath. I now had a problem, both the husband and 'arry were little men, it was obvious we were not going to get the lady out the bath alone. We had to get the fire lads there. However, she adamantly said she would not allow it. No matter what I said she would die before letting the firemen in; in view of the situation, she was probably right about dying as well. I got on the radio and requested the attendance of her doctor and a couple of coppers. The doctor was on his rounds, but in a few minutes the law arrived in the form of two big lads in a patrol car.

We worked out a plan of getting her out. The two coppers and I stood in a line by the bath and pushed our hands between her and the sides of the bath shoving in a blanket as we did so, getting it between her and the smooth bath. It was a long and slow job, and also a wet one, but at last we had a blanket down one side, under her and up the other. There was only just enough room for the three of us to stand side by side, so the lift was quite a struggle. After lots of heaving, tugging and effort, with a horrible slurping noise we rolled her out and onto the floor. The lady was relived and at once started to perk up. Wrapping our now free patient in dry blankets we placed her onto our little chair, and with the help of the law we carried her downstairs. Once we had her into the ambulance and onto the stretcher, despite her protestations, we took her to the hospital for a check-up. It was not the sort of job we got very often for which I was very grateful.

Only a short time after that job, we had another call involving a bathroom. This time it was a lot easier to handle. The lady had gone to the shop and left her husband soaking in the tub with a book. She had returned and after some time had shouted to him that she had made a cup of tea. Receiving no reply she had taken it up. She was a little surprised to find the door locked for he did not usually bother. She knocked and got no reply. By this time the wife was beginning to become concerned. She shouted and banged on the door. There was nothing but silence from the room. He must have collapsed. She panicked, envisaging him unconscious in the bath, perhaps he had collapsed, slipped into the water and drowned. She dialled 999 and shouted for an ambulance. We were on station and arrived on scene within two minutes. It took a few more minutes to calm down the now hysterical wife and find out what had happened. As soon as we made out what she was trying to say we rushed up to the bathroom door. Knocking and shouting had no effect. It was obvious he was unconscious and we had to get into him. In a situation like that on the TV, the hero would throw his shoulder at the door and burst into the room. I had long since learned that this doesn't happen in real life, all it achieves is a bruised shoulder! I asked the wife if they had a big hammer. She said yes, and rushed out, returning a few moments later with the type of hammer you might use crack toffee! Bert went to the vehicle and used the radio to request the fire service. I meanwhile had a look outside to see if there was any means of getting in through the window. It was of course high and in the centre of a blank wall. We returned to the solid bathroom door.

We heard the two-tone horns of the fire brigade as they turned out of their station; for a retained crew they were really on the ball. Within minutes they were at the house and I was explaining to the Sub-Officer what was required. He quickly told two of his crew to get a ladder up to the window, and, carrying a big axe, he followed me to the bathroom door.

"No problem" he said and squared himself to the door, measuring the swing he needed. "Stand well back, give me room…" he instructed as he lifted the axe.

At that point, a small voice asked what was going on. The Sub told the fellow to stand back.

"I'm damned if I will," the voice said, "why are you in my house and why are you chopping my bathroom door down?"

We all turned and looked at the man. The woman screamed and threw her arms around him. The man explained that after finishing his bath he had gone to the shop. He was most surprised to find an ambulance and fire engine outside his house when he returned!

We were all feeling very pleased with the situation when we heard a shattering of glass. A voice from the other side of the door shouted.

"We've got in. There's no one in here but the towel rail has dropped and jammed the door."

Fortunately, the husband took his smashed window in good part and we all went home.

We had another experience with the Fire Service and bathrooms a year or so later. On that occasion it was our turn to look foolish.

We were at Ambulance Headquarters, having taken a patient to the nearby hospital. We had called with the sole intention of seeing what gossip we could glean and what we could scrounge in the way of spare kit or equipment. Having had no luck with either, we were about to leave just as the emergency buzzer went and an emergency call came in. The Controller asked if we could cover it, and showed us the location on the large wall map. It was easy for us to find, so we offered to attend. The caller said it was a report of an old lady collapsed in her home. Rob swung the vehicle out of the yard and with beacon flashing and horns making enough noise to waken the dead, we made our way down the road to the incident.

We were always a little apprehensive when covering an emergency in a strange town in case we got lost – there is nothing more embarrassing than having to back out of a cul-de-sac into which you have rushed with everything blazing! As we turned into the road, we at once spotted an agitated old gent, waving frantically to attract our attention. We had obviously reached our destination. Pulling up outside the house I jumped out to attend to him. Like most people at an incident, and especially the old, the man was in a state of panic and shock. I did my best to calm him down as we tried to find out what was involved and, more to the point, where the patient was.

I have been to many calls to find that someone other than the patient has collapsed in their excitement, and two patients makes things far more complicated. After what seemed an age, we gleaned that his wife had collapsed in the bathroom upstairs.

We went into the terraced house, up the stairs and found the bathroom facing us. The top panel of the door was frosted glass and through it I could see the form of an old person lying on the floor. I tapped on the door and called out to her, she did not move. Constant knocking and calls, from both us, and her husband, evoked no response, and I began to fear the worst. We were in a 'no-win situation'. She was unconscious and could do nothing to help herself, but we could not get in to help her. We could see that she was lying between the door and the side of the bath, thus preventing us from pushing the door open. She was also too near the door to allow us to break the glass, in case some fell on her and did her further injury.

We had to get help, and in a case like this, as quickly as we could. I sent Rob down to the radio to request help; we needed the fire service. Meanwhile, I did my best to try to talk to the old lady and also to calm her husband, who was now greatly agitated and entering a state of shock. I was quickly getting into the position of having to treat two patients. Whilst giving the outward impression of calm, I was hoping desperately that a fire crew would soon arrive and let me get to my patient. Rob returned and said they were on the way and I delightedly breathed a sigh of relief.

I was even more pleased when I heard the sound of the fire appliance pulling up outside. Apart from their horns to tell of their approach, firemen always seem to have the radio loudly transmitting to the whole of the street, which sometimes can be very distracting, but that day it was music to my ears. Within moments, I heard the sound of heavy boots on the stairs and a Sub-Officer and fireman arrived at my side. They were a full time professional crew and would soon get me to my patient. I explained the problem, and stepped back to let them to the door. The Sub knocked on the door and shouted through the glass to the old lady.

"Are you all right pet?" Imagine my surprise when I heard a soft weak voice say yes. He half turned and grinned at me, then put his face back to the glass.

"Can you hear me?"

Again the soft yes.

"Can you move so that we can get into the door?"

With that, she said yes again and moved!

We all walked in.

I don't think I have ever felt such an idiot!

CHAPTER TWENTY NINE

Helping the Police

The play had just started on the 'box'. It was one of the best series they had put on for years, and tonight was the final episode; I had been looking forward to it all week. The telephone rang and I picked it up with a groan – of course, it was Control with a job.

"Aw give it to some other crew, I've had a rotten day."

I could almost see him grin at the other end of the line, "Can't mate, it's at your local nick."

I growled to the controller to pass the details. I could tell he was enjoying himself!

"You'll like this one mate, it's a local yobbo, he's been in a punch up and flattened a couple of coppers. Now he has to go to the County, ASP."

I couldn't understand this situation.

"If he's in the nick, why don't the law take him in a van?"

I was told he had a broken leg, so muttering loudly, I reached for my coat.

I was on standby with 'Old 'arry'. Harry was a nice enough old bloke and a first class First Aider. He'd been a member of the Service as an Auxiliary since it started… a veritable 'salt of the earth'. The problem was, Harry was a tiny, nervous chap, thin as a rail and getting on in years. He was not exactly my first choice for a crewmate when dealing with a fellow who had just laid out two coppers!

CALL AN AMBULANCE! • 227

Still it was our job and we had to get on with it. We met at the station and when I told my colleague what we had in store, his Adam's apple began to bob up and down in panic and his eyes blinked non-stop behind his owl-like specs. We got the bus out and drove to the Police Station, it was only around the corner. The town was a nice quiet little place, and we rarely had any trouble; it was the sort of place where people read about punch-ups in bigger towns and tut-tutted. Tonight, the normally quiet police station was alive with cars and lights. Parking in front and entering, I could not help but notice that 'Old 'arry' had not said a lot, and kept well behind me.

The front office was full. Although only a small room, it was full of coppers, all chattering, shouting and laughing loudly. Of course, 'Nosey Parker' was there. Nosey was the sergeant, the same one who'd taken me on my driving test years before. Nosey was a great character, one of the 'old school' of coppers. He looked every bit the old time copper: big, fat, red faced, bald and near to retirement. His nickname was understandable when you saw him. Nosey had been involved in a punch up as a young bobby, and what with his injury and his liking for a pint, his large, bulbous nose was the feature you noticed first – a great red thing, glowing like a beacon, that covered most of his equally red, fleshy face. To make the thing even more noticeable, it was supported by a magnificent sweeping moustache. As soon as Nosey saw us, his features creased into a broad grin. As he beckoned to us, he banged on the desk. Silence fell as the assembled constabulary turned to study us.

"Come on in lads! By gum I'm right pleased ter see you, you're just what we need right now."

I was immediately suspicious. No-one ever looked that pleased to see us unless there was a reason! Silence fell whilst Nosey told us the full story. It seemed the patient was a soldier, a 'Para', who had met a local girl on his last leave and become attached. As soon as Nosey mentioned her name I groaned. The 'lady' in question was very well known as the 'town bike', and I guessed the rest of the tale before Nosey had finished speaking. The squaddie had returned, full of love and lust, only to find his beloved 'out on the town'. He had searched the pubs and had eventually found his beloved, extremely 'well oiled' and in the arms of a cattle truck driver, about to test the warmth of the straw in his truck. Words had been exchanged and a fight had, of course developed, naturally with the rest of the pub joining in. The local bobby had happened to be cycling past, and having taken one look, called for help and waited until the 'heavy mob' arrived.

It seemed the young soldier was a dab-hand with his fists, with the result that two coppers and the truck driver had already been taken to the County hospital in a Police van as walking wounded. I bit my tongue and didn't ask why they were trying to put me out of work.

"So what do you want us for Nosey? Ain't you got any more vans with nothing to do?" I enquired with a straight face.

Nosey pointedly ignored my sarcasm and beamed broadly while the other coppers shuffled their feet.

"Well, as the lads 'ere wus puttin him into the cell, chummy aimed a kick at Eric's weddin' tackle. Now Eric, being pretty nimble 'cause of his ballroom dancin' leapt arta the way and chummy kicks bleedin wall."

Nosey tapped the painted bricks with his hand.

"Them Victorians wot built this ere nick knew as 'ow ter do it so as it wern't ter fall down ... built as solid as one of them brick shit houses. Owd Doc Rider reckons chummy bust his toes, so we thought about you lads and ow yer orta give 'im a bit of tender luvvin care."

"Thank you very much! I said, sarcastically.

Nosey again ignored me.

"Right oh..." I said with a sigh, "...let the dog see the rabbit! Lets have a look at him and then we'll take him away." I was not feeling half as brave as I sounded. If this guy had caused as much damage as they said he had, I didn't feel too keen about getting close to him. We all crowded out into the passage and down to the cell door.

Nosey had been right about the station being built to last, it must have been built before they started to think about costs. The wall of the cell was about two feet thick, making the doorway a small, narrow tunnel. I went in and looked at the patient laid on the narrow bed. They were right about his size as well, he was certainly a big fella. Chummy scowled at me and my friendly "How do... Ambulance" made little difference to his expression. I said I had to look at his foot and he said nothing, just lay there looking at me. The toes were well and truly fractured, there was no way could he walk.

In those days ambulancemen were accepted as neutral. We could go into fights and wild sessions, and whilst they would continue the punch up around us, they all ignored us, knowing we were trying to help. I regret to say that this no longer applies to the modern crews who are now all too often targets for violence. We always tried to establish a rapport with everyone, but this guy chose to ignore any attempts at friendship. I left him on the bed and returned to Nosey.

"The only way we'll be able to get him out of there is by carrying him out on a carry sheet. I'll need some of your lads to give us a lift".

The coppers nodded acceptance and waited until we got organised. With the ambulance backed up to the doors of the nick, I explained to the coppers how we would do the lift and what I wanted them to do. Obediently, they let me take charge. Old 'arry and I entered the cell and although the patient refused to speak, he listened to me whilst I explained what we were going to do. After strapping up his foot, the next stage of the removal entailed us rolling the canvas carry sheet and easing it under him. We then rolled our patient from side to side until the sheet was underneath him. Just like that! The sheet had handles down each side which would allow the patient to be carried out and into the waiting ambulance. Three hefty coppers crowded into the cell with us and, getting hold of the handles we stood in a line by the bed. At my command, we lifted together so that the soldier was supported in a level line. We then shuffled sideways out of the cell and through the narrow doorway.

It was whilst pushed tightly against our patient in the cell door that I glanced down and looked into the man's eyes. Those eyes were full of pure hatred, and more to the point his clenched fist was in line with my nose! I had a moment of panic, thinking that if he lashed out I could end up with a hooter just like Nosey! Needless to say, I was pleased when we reached the vehicle. I was also pleased when Nosey allocated two big bobbies to act as escorts for the journey. We did, however, protest when he told one of them to put cuffs on the patient. This guy may have been difficult, and he was their prisoner, but he was my patient in my ambulance. I was a little surprised when I won. Naturally, Harry drove to the hospital, in fact he was behind the wheel before I could say anything! Truth to tell, he would not have been a lot of use in the back, but I was not too sure of myself being a lot of use either! We sat in a line watching the patient, who said not a word for the whole of the half-hour journey. We didn't have a single bad moment for the whole of the run, but I was not sorry when I saw the lights of the lodge as we drove into County Hospital.

It would have been a completely uneventful episode had it not been for Old 'arry. It was not his fault, it was just that he didn't think, and as an ambulanceman thinking can be the most important bit! We sat in our line and waited until he positioned and parked the ambulance. Fetching the trolley 'arry opened the doors. I told the law to climb out and as they did 'arry pulled the catch at the end of the stretcher to release it. The stretcher would then be free to slide part way out on a runner which would enable me to take the head end. As 'arry leaned across the foot of the patient to reach the catch, the last copper slipped on the step, and as he did he nudged 'arry, who lost his footing and dropped onto the patient's injured foot.

The silent soldier gave a bellow of pain, and kicked 'arry in the chest with his good foot. It would have been a blow felt by most men, but with 'arry being so small and light, that kick propelled him straight out of the ambulance and after a short but graceful flight, into a small heap on the ground. It all happened so quickly the police naturally thought that the prisoner was attempting to escape. Both coppers leapt back into the ambulance and onto the patient. A wild scuffle immediately developed: arms, legs, blankets, effin and blindin, with poor old 'arry lying on the ground moaning. All the time I was trying to steady the patient's leg so that he did not do any more damage to himself. All was utter chaos until suddenly a voice bellowed, "Stop this noise in my department at once!"

We froze. Silence immediately descended. We shamefacedly sorted ourselves out and, releasing the stretcher, meekly followed the Nursing Sister into Casualty.

Throughout my years in the Ambulance Service, I never ceased to marvel at how much authority an experienced Nursing Sister could have over people!

CHAPTER THIRTY

Horses for Courses

I have never been one for horses. I expect they are all right if you like them, but I always found they had big feet, always seeming intent on treading on mine. I liked to watch the hunt when it was out, but only from a safe distance, and apart from the odd times when we received a call to go and pick up a rider, with me always ensuring that someone kept an eye on the horse whilst I was working on my patient, I never went too near them.

Apart from being part of a syndicate on the pools at work, I have never been a gambler either, so when I moved, the fact that the town had a racecourse meant nothing to me. Smithy was excited though. Smithy considered himself to be an expert on form, spending hours reading papers, looking at racing books and doing complicated sums on the back of fag packets. He would also spend a lot of time on the telephone to bookmakers, speaking a strange language of 'Yankees', 'doubles' and 'accumulators'. We suspected that Smithy never won much, but he was certainly an addict. When Smithy discovered where I had been posted, he gave me strict instructions to let him have any tips I received from 'those in the know'. However, I never found out who 'those in the know' were, and forgot all about his request. Apart from seeing the racecourse as we passed it from time to time and knowing men who worked on it, we had little contact with the racing fraternity. However, on race days, the town became unbelievably busy, and the racecourse was usually packed. I went with my wife once, but we didn't get the bug and lost interest, but the course did add a little colour to our lives.

The three of us had got into the habit of having a drink after work on a Friday evening; it was the only night none of us was on standby. At exactly six o' clock we would all go across the road from the station and into the Swan. It could not be classed as a 'session', because we had one round each then went home; Rob always had strict instructions from his missus as to what time he had to be home for his tea. It was by chance, whilst in that salubrious establishment one evening, that we met a set of little guys in the bar. It transpired that they were 'stable boys', although they all seemed very old to be called boys. During the course of conversation, we discovered that they always spent the night before a race at the Swan whereas the jockeys used the Wheatsheaf and the toffs used the Crown. I had not realised such a strict hierarchy existed amongst the racing fraternity. We were about to go, when I remembered Smithy's words, and asked if they had a tip. One little man winked broadly and whispered. "Poot a fair bit on them 'osses fra a weel known brewery."

We left the pub in great excitement. Rob said he'd not dare risk it, but Bert said the little Jock obviously knew a lot about racecourses, so he would have a quid on it. I told my wife about our tip during tea and, rather than tell Smithy, decided we would keep it to ourselves and risk a bet in the morning. We studied the morning paper and agreed we would lash out and risk five shillings (25 pence) on each horse. I went off to the betting shop and placed my bet. The man asked me if I wanted it 'on the nose'. I hadn't a clue what he was talking about but, not wishing to sound ignorant, I said yes. It was only later that I found I should have had it as a 'place'.

Settling in front of the TV, we watched our first race with great interest. 'Our' horse stayed at the front but came second. I was told off for getting the bet wrong! Our other horse was running in the next race but one. By now we were both excited; the racing bug had finally got to us. The race started at last and although we had definitely seen it in the line up it was not mentioned again. It must have got bored and gone home! The racing bug quickly left us. We couldn't afford to chuck ten shillings away like that!

Apart from that one episode of gambling, I lost interest in race days. My only feelings were those of annoyance when called out and having to fight through race day traffic to get to a job. Only rarely were we called to the racecourse on a race day. The officials employed stewards who looked after any minor injuries on the course, and we were only called if a patient had to go to hospital. Apart from being aware that the local voluntary aid society wanted to take on the role of first aid on the course, it was of no interest to us.

It was a big meeting on the day we had a call to take a jockey, who had had a bad fall, into hospital. I lived on the road next to the course and stood at the gate enjoying the sun as I waited for Rob to collect me. As we drove down to the course, he mentioned that the row about who was to do first aid there was hotting up again. I took little interest. We arrived and wove our way slowly through the crowds to the 'first aid station' – a rather gracious title for a small wooden hut. We walked in and sensed at once a hostile atmosphere. Dr Davies, the local GP, was standing by the patient and looking very cross. Three stewards were standing at the feet of the patient, each looking rather uncomfortable and somewhat shifty. An important-looking man in a smart suit and bowler hat, with a pair of binoculars hanging around his neck, stood in the corner. On the bench in the centre of the room lay the jockey, still dressed in brightly coloured racing silks. A long wooden splint was tied to his right leg by two triangular bandages, which did not look very effective or very neat. Dr Davies spoke in a soft voice.

"This gentleman has a fracture of the left lower leg". I looked at Rob and he looked at me. Whilst we didn't know a lot, we did know that a splint was used on the side of the injury. We also knew a lower leg fracture needed more than two bandages. I looked at Rob.

"We'll get the stretcher mate."

We returned to our vehicle.

"What had happened?" was the question on both our lips. I took command, as L/A it was my responsibility.

"Look Rob, there's politics here regarding this lot, and we're not getting involved. If Davies wants the guy in, we'll load him and sort him out in the back of the ambulance."

Rob, never wishing to fall out with anyone, quickly agreed.

We re-entered the room with the stretcher, carefully loaded the patient onto it, covered him with a blanket and took him out to the ambulance. All the time there was a strange silence in the first aid room.

In the ambulance, my questions and checks confirmed the patient had a fracture of the lower left leg; his right leg was fine. We treated him accordingly, made him comfortable, and then set off for the hospital. On the journey, I tried to find out why the jockey had had a splint on his uninjured leg, but he had no idea. It was certainly beyond us, and discussed every possible reason we could think of on our return run.

We decided we had better not mention it, and quickly forgot all about the incident.

The following week, driving through town, we saw Dr Davies. He flagged us down, and his opening words took us by surprise.

"You are a couple of prize prats!"

We looked at the Doctor in amazement; hurt and surprised. He carefully explained.

"I've been at that course for years, arguing to get a better standard of first-aid cover. At last when I think I've won, when I have a jockey who has obviously been treated incorrectly, when I have the Clerk of the course on my side, I send for the elite. I call for the County Ambulance Service. I said to the idiot stewards, 'Stand back and watch how these lads deal with a patient – they are the experts'."

The Doctor paused, eyes flickering between us. Rob had coloured up and I guessed what he was going to say next.

"Then you two come in and stand there like a couple of spare dicks at a wedding. You pick him up without a word and like a couple of prats just calmly take him away!"

There was not a great deal we could say...

CHAPTER THIRTY ONE

The Dog

We never thought a lot about politics, we never thought much about the NHS. We worked in hospitals every day and knew a lot of people, but they were nothing to do with us, because we were Council staff – the NHS were different. So it came as a shock one day to discover that we were going to be taken over by them!

It was Rob who mentioned it first. It was early one evening and we were all on station and washing the vehicles down in the yard.

"Ere mate, I was in the King's last night and Chalky White said we were going to be taken over by the NHS in the review. What was he on about?"

Bert threw the wash leather at him.

"Shurrup yer silly old sod, you're just like an old woman listening to gossip. Chalky White knows less about the NHS than I do and that's sod all. How's he know owt about it, he's only a milkman?"

The banter continued until we went home, it was just a normal evening. I had finished my tea and was glancing through the local rag when I caught the headline about the change in the County boundary. I knew they were messing about and changing things but how could they have a new County taking over a bit of ours? It was silly, we'd always covered that bit, how could it become part of a new Local Authority? I turned the page, pleased I'd moved as it wouldn't affect me.

I was on the 'sitting bus' that week and took the usual patients into the hospital near to our parent station. I called them and said I was coming down with my returns and to collect stores. I was checking the items I wanted with the L/A, when the Fairy Queen called me into his office and queried a point regarding some figures on a petrol return. We sorted the problem and started to talk about a number of subjects, and as we chatted, he shocked me by asking if I was going to stay or move back to my old station. I suddenly realised that I was not as well informed as I had thought. Without letting on about my ignorance of the developing situation, I let him talk. It was clear that 1974 was going to have an enormous effect upon us all. The local government boundary changes were to coincide with a number of changes within the NHS, the most important one being that the Ambulance Services were being passed over to the NHS instead of remaining under Local Council control. The news came as a shock, and for the first time in my life I realised that decisions made by government did affect me! Not only were boundaries to be changed but amalgamations and take-overs were to be the order of the day. Our County Service was to combine with three others. I was horrified; I didn't like the idea at all. Like most people, I didn't welcome change and wanted things to stay as they were. It was only as I was leaving that Quentin said something which made me think twice.

"This should be eggs and bacon for you dear, I bet your ever so excited aren't you?"

I looked at him. At times our Station Officer did talk like a prat. What had I got to be excited about? Whatever was he going on about?

"Well", I said, "I may be, or then again I may not be, I'll have to keep my eye on things won't I."

'If in doubt, play your hand close to your chest' seemed the right policy; I had no idea what he was going on about, but I was sure as hell not going to let on. As I had hoped, he fell for my noncommittal line. He grinned.

"Stop messing me about Sweetheart! I'll bet as soon as you saw the proposals for the amalgamation your active little mind started to work non stop, sorting out all the chances of you getting a white shirt and pips out of the re-organisation."

I gave Quentin one of my knowing looks and left before he had chance to realise he was far beyond me. Blimey! I'd never thought about promotion. Could it be there was going to be a bit of movement and a vacancy. That promotion bug was beginning to bite again!

As plans began to formulate and the scale of change became apparent, I started to take a greater interest in the surrounding Services. Most of our journeys were into the City Hospital, which was served by a small City Service. An adjoining Service, with which we were to merge, also took patients into the City hospitals. We, of course, knew and met all the road staff of both Services. Apart from knowing that the City had few officers, I knew little about the County's situation. I very quickly made it my business to find out more. In the main, all the officers seemed old and not interested in promotion. Although our Service was pretty basic, it seemed that the others were worse off than we were. It appeared that 'Taff' our CAO had the most chance of taking over the 'new' Service. I began to feel rather confident that things could be going my way, and I'm sure that I became the only person to be looking forward to the coming changes.

For the first time, but certainly not the last, I started to study form and competition in the promotion stakes. As part of this plan I started to study the potential challenge from the other Services. Although I didn't know it at the time, it was to be the start of my progression through the ranks within a number of Ambulance Services. It was during this period that I heard the following classic tale of trying hard but getting it wrong...

"Would you put the cat out mister."

"Could you make sure the door is locked, and check I turned the gas off please love."

It was all part and parcel of the job to look after our patients welfare in addition to their ambulance care, especially the elderly, when going for treatment. We were well aware that many of our elderly patients saw no one from when we dropped them off until we collected them again days later. It was this extra touch of care and attention which one day caused a great deal of embarrassment to a couple of ambulance crew from the City, as they rather shamefacedly related to us at the tea bar one morning. Maggie and Pauline worked as a day crew. The City employed both emergency shift staff and day crews for non emergency details. They were also one of the first to employ women, about which we were all a little sceptical, but had to grudgingly admit they did a good job. I'm sure Pauline would not take offence if I said she was the motherly kind. Nothing was too much trouble and she had the knack of making each person feel that little bit special. Whilst everyone had compassion towards their patients, she had that little bit extra. On the day in question they were on an outpatient run in the City, in and out of estates and hospitals, picking up and dropping off, trying all the time to get patients in on time and get them home again without too much delay. It was mid morning when they picked up a patient new to them.

Mr Black was in his mid-fifties and lived alone. He had recently had a leg amputated and was confined to a wheelchair. Pauline fussed around Mr Black ensuring he was well wrapped up against the cold wind. When satisfied, they wheeled him out in his own chair and placed him in the ambulance. Maggie was closing the ambulance doors and Pauline was about to take his chair back to the house when he called to her, asking her to make sure the dog was not left out as she was on heat. As instructed, Pauline shooed the dog in. It was so cold the animal took little persuading and rushed into the house and warmth. Locking the door she passed the keys to Mr Black assuring all was well and safe.

It was much later in the day when Mr Black's treatment was finished and he was ready for home. Maggie and Pauline were detailed to return him, so they met again. When they arrived back at his home they took him from the ambulance to his door on their carry chair. At the door he requested they help him stand on his one leg and said he could hop in when the door was opened. With Mr Black's arm around their shoulders, Maggie unlocked the door. As soon as he pushed it open, a large, black mongrel dog pushed past them and ran down the street. The effect of seeing the dog was like an electric shock to the patient. He gave a strangled scream and uttered a string of oaths and curses. At the same time he swung on the shoulders of the crew whilst he attempted, unsuccessfully, to kick the dog with the amputated leg. Needless to say the dog was away like a shot.

The ambulance crew were amazed at the change in their patient and quickly carried the distraught man into his house and sat him in his chair. Mr Black was almost in tears, red faced, and uttering moans and wails of distress. They did their best to calm him down, very well aware that in his condition, his anxiety could bring on a stroke or a heart attack.

They had almost brought Mr Black back to a stable condition when Maggie felt something by her side. She looked down and saw a dog. It was a Golden Labrador, an obviously well cared-for, pedigree animal. The dog that had caused such distress to Mr Black had been a scruffy nondescript black thing. Maggie looked down again at the dog. She may have imagined it, but the dog seemed to have a very satisfied expression on its face.

Maggie caught Pauline's eye and inclined her head toward the dog. The look on her face was a picture. At that point the patient spoke.

"How on earth did that damn thing manage to get in? It's been trying to get at Floss since she came on heat last week. It'll have ruined her."

Pauline coloured up and gulped. Her mouth opened and closed a number of times. Her normally placid and relaxed attitude melted.

"Mr B… B… Black," she stuttered, "you remember when we collected you and you told me to make sure the dog was in…"

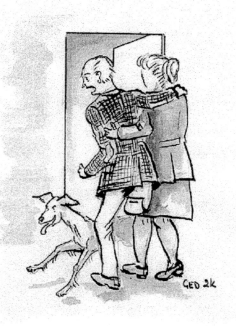

Also published by Woodfield...
The following titles are all available in our unique high-quality softback format

RAF HUMOUR
Bawdy Ballads & Dirty Ditties of the RAF – A huge collection of the bawdy songs and rude recitations beloved by RAF personnel in WW2. Certain to amuse any RAF veteran. Uncensored – so strictly adults only! *"Not for the frail, the frightfully posh or proper gels – but great fun for everyone else!"* **£9.95**

Upside Down Nothing on the Clock – Dozens of jokes and anecdotes contributed by RAF personnel from AC2s to the top brass... still one of our best sellers. *"Highly enjoyable."* **£6.00**

Upside Down Again! – Our second great collection of RAF jokes, funny stories and anecdotes – a great gift for those with a high-flying sense of humour! *"Very funny indeed."* **£6.00**

Was It Like This For You? – A feast of humorous reminiscences & cartoons depicting the more comical aspects of life in the RAF. *"Will bring back many happy memories. Highly recommended."* **£6.00**

MILITARY MEMOIRS & HISTORIES – THE POST-WAR PERIOD
I Have Control... Former RAF Parachute instructor **Edward Cartner** humorously recalls the many mishaps, blunders and faux-pas of his military career. *Superb writing; very amusing indeed.* **£9.95**

Korea: We Lived They Died Former soldier with Duke of Wellington's Regt **Alan Carter** reveals the appalling truth of front-line life for British troops in this now forgotten war. *Very funny in places too.* **£9.95**

Meteor Eject! Former 257 Sqn pilot [1950s] **Nick Carter** recalls the early days of RAF jets and his many adventures flying Meteors, including one very lucky escape via a Mk.2 Martin-Baker ejector seat... **£9.95**

Pluck Under Fire Eventful Korean War experiences of **John Pluck** with the Middlesex Regiment. **£9.95**

Return to Gan • Michael Butler's light-hearted account of life at RAF Gan in 1960 and the founding of 'Radio Gan'. *Will delight those who also served at this remote RAF outpost in the Indian Ocean.* **£12.00**

Tread Lightly into Danger • Bomb-disposal expert **Anthony Charlwood**'s experiences in some of the world's most dangerous hotspots (Kuwait, Iraq, Lebanon, Somalia, etc) over the last 30 years. **£9.95**

The Spice of Flight • Former RAF pilot **Richard Pike** delivers a fascinating account of flying Lightnings, Phantoms and later helicopters with 56, 43(F) & 19 Sqns in the RAF of the 1960s & 70s. **£9.95**

Flying the Waves • **Richard Pike** describes his eventful second career as a commercial helicopter pilot, which involved him in many Coastguard Air/Sea Rescue operations in the Shetlands and North Sea. **£9.95**

MILITARY MEMOIRS & HISTORIES – WORLD WAR 1 & 2
2297: A POW's Story • Taken prisoner at Dunkirk, **John Lawrence** spent 5 years as a POW at Lamsdorf, Jagendorf, Posen and elsewhere. *"A very interesting & delightfully illustrated account of his experiences."* **£6.00**

A Bird Over Berlin Former Lancaster pilot with 61 Sqn, **Tony Bird DFC** tells a remarkable tale of survival against the odds during raids on the German capital & as a POW. *"An incredible-but-true sequence of events."* **£9.95**

A Journey from Blandford The wartime exploits of motorcycle dispatch rider **B.A. Jones** began at Blandford Camp in Dorset but took him to Dunkirk, the Middle East, D-Day and beyond... **£9.95**

A Lighter Shade of Blue A former Radar Operator **Reg O'Neil** recalls his WW2 service in Malta and Italy with 16004 AMES – a front-line mobile radar unit. *'Interesting, informative and amusing.'* **£9.95**

A Shillingsworth of Promises Delightfully funny and ribald memoirs of **Fred Hitchcock** recalling his years as an RAF airman during the war and later amusing escapades in the UK and Egypt. *A very entertaining read.* **£9.95**

Beaufighters BOAC & Me – WW2 Beaufighter navigator **Sam Wright** served a full tour with 254 Sqn and was later seconded to BOAC on early postwar overseas routes. *'Captures the spirit of the Beaufighter'* **£9.95**

Coastal Command Pilot Former Hudson pilot **Ted Rayner**'s outstanding account of his unusual WW2 Coastal Command experiences, flying in the Arctic from bases in Iceland and Greenland. **£9.95**

Cyril Wild: The Tall Man Who Never Slept – **James Bradley**'s biography of a remarkable Japanese-speaking British Army officer who helped many POWs survive on the infamous Burma railway. **£9.95**

Desert War Diary by **John Walton** Diary and photos recording the activities of the Hurricanes and personnel of 213 Squadron during WW2 in Cyprus and Egypt. *"Informative and entertaining."* **£9.95**

From Fiji to Balkan Skies Spitfire/Mustang pilot **Dennis McCaig** recalls eventful WW2 operations over the Adriatic/Balkans with 249 Sqn in 43/44. *'A rip-roaring real-life adventure, splendidly written.'* **£9.95**

From Horses to Chieftains – Long-serving Army veteran **Richard Napier** recalls an eventful Army career that began with a cavalry regiment in 1935; took in El Alamein & D-Day and ended in the 1960s. **£9.95**

Get Some In! The many wartime adventures of **Mervyn Base**, a WW2 RAF Bomb Disposal expert **£9.95**

Just a Survivor Former Lancaster navigator **Phil Potts** tells his remarkable tale of survival against the odds in the air with 103 Sqn and later as a POW. *'An enlightening and well written account.'* **£9.95**

Memoirs of a 'Goldfish' • The eventful wartime memoirs of former 115 Sqn Wellington pilot **Jim Burtt-Smith**, now president of the Goldfish Club - exclusively for aviators who have force-landed into water. **£9.95**

No Brylcreem, No Medals – RAF MT driver **Jack Hambleton** 's splendid account of his wartime escapades in England, Shetlands & Middle East blends comic/tragic aspects of war in uniquely entertaining way. **£8.00**

Nobody's Hero • Former RAF Policeman **Bernard Hart-Hallam**'s extraordinary adventures with 2TAF Security Section on D-Day and beyond in France, Belgium & Germany. *"Unique and frequently surprising."* **£9.95**

Once a Cameron Highlander • This biog of Robert Burns, who, at 104 was the oldest survivor of the Battle of the Somme; takes in his WW1 experiences, later life in showbusiness and celebrity status as a centenarian. **£9.95**

Operation Pharos • **Ken Rosam** tells the story of the RAF's secret bomber base/staging post on the Cocos Keeling islands during WW2 and of many operations from there. *'A fascinating slice of RAF history.'* **£9.95**

Over Hell & High Water • WW2 navigator **Les Parsons** survived 31 ops on Lancasters with 622 Sqn, then went on to fly Liberators in Far East with 99 Sqn. *'An exceptional tale of 'double jeopardy'.* **£9.95**

Pacifist to Glider Pilot • The son of Plymouth Brethren parents, **Alec Waldron** renounced their pacifism and went on to pilot gliders with the Glider Pilot Regiment at both Sicily & Arnhem. *Excellent photos.* **£9.95**

Pathfinder Force Balkans – Pathfinder F/Engineer **Geoff Curtis** saw action over Germany & Italy before baling out over Hungary. He was a POW in Komarno, Stalags 17a & 17b. *'An amazing catalogue of adventures.'* **£9.95**

Per Ardua Pro Patria • Humour and tragedy are interwoven in these unassuming autobiographical observations of **Dennis Wiltshire**, a former Lancaster Flight Engineer who later worked for NASA. **£9.95**

Ploughs, Planes & Palliasses • Entertaining recollections of RAF pilot **Percy Carruthers**, who flew Baltimores in Egypt with 223 Squadron and was taken a POW at Stalag Luft 1 & 6. **£9.95**

RAF/UXB The Story of RAF Bomb Disposal • Stories contributed by wartime RAF BD veterans that will surprise and educate the uninitiated. *"Amazing stories of very brave men."* **£9.95**

Railway to Runway • Wartime diary & letters of Halifax Observer **Leslie Harris** – killed in action with 76 Sqn in 1943 – poignantly capture the spirit of the wartime RAF in the words of a 20-year-old airman. **£9.95**

Seletar Crowning Glory • The history of the RAF base in Singapore from its earliest beginnings, through the golden era of the flying-boats, its capture in WW2 and on to its closure in the 1970s. **£15.00**

The RAF & Me • Former Stirling navigator **Gordon Frost** recalls ops with 570 Sqn from RAF Harwell, including 'Market-Garden' 'Varsity' and others. *'A salute to the mighty Stirling and its valiant crews.'* **£9.95**

Training for Triumph • **Tom Docherty**'s very thorough account of the amazing achievement of RAF Training Command, who trained over 90,000 aircrew during World War 2. *'An impressively detailed book.'* **£12.00**

Un Grand Bordel • Geoffrey French relates air-gunner **Norman Lee**'s amazing real-life adventures with the French Maquis (Secret Army) after being shot down over Europe. *"Frequently funny and highly eventful."* **£9.95**

UXB Vol 2 More unusual and gripping tales of bomb disposal in WW2 and after. **£9.95**

Wot! No Engines? • Alan Cooper tells the story of military gliders in general and the RAF glider pilots who served on Operation Varsity in 1945 in particular. A very large and impressive book with many photos. **£18.00**

While Others Slept • Former Hampden navigator **Eric Woods** tells the story of Bomber Command's early years and how he completed a tour of duty with 144 Squadron. *'Full of valuable historical detail.'* **£9.95**

WOMEN & WORLD WAR TWO

A WAAF at War • Former MT driver **Diana Lindo**'s charming evocation of life in the WAAF will bring back happy memories to all those who also served in World War 2. *"Nostalgic and good-natured."* **£9.95**

Corduroy Days • Warm-hearted and amusing recollections of **Josephine Duggan-Rees**'s wartime years spent as a Land Girl on farms in the New Forest area. *"Funny, nostalgic and very well written."* **£9.95**

Ernie • **Celia Savage**'s quest to discover the truth about the death of her father, an RAF Halifax navigator with 149 Sqn, who died in WW2 when she was just 6 years old. *"A real-life detective story."* **£9.95**

In My Father's Footsteps • **Pat Bienkowski**'s moving account of her trip to Singapore & Thailand to visit the places where her father and uncle were both POW's during WW2. **£9.95**

Lambs in Blue • **Rebecca Barnett**'s revealing account of the wartime lives and loves of a group of WAAFs posted to the tropical paradise of Ceylon. *'A highly congenial WW2 chronicle."* **£9.95**

Radar Days • Delightful evocation of life in the wartime WAAF by former Radar Operator **Gwen Arnold**, who served at Bawdsey Manor RDF Station, Suffolk. *"Amusing, charming and affectionate."* **£9.95**

Searching in the Dark The amusing wartime diary of **Peggy Butler** a WAAF radar operator 1942-1946 – written when she was just 19 yrs old and serving at Bawdsey RDF station in Suffolk **£9.95**

MEMOIRS & HISTORIES – NON-MILITARY

20th CenturyFarmers Boy • Sussex farmer **Nick Adames** looks back on a century of rural change and what it has meant to his own family and the county they have farmed in for 400 years. **£9.95**

Call an Ambulance! • former ambulance driver **Alan Crosskill** recalls a number of light-hearted episodes from his eventful career in the 1960s/70s. 'Very amusing and entertaining'. **£9.95**

Harry – An Evacuee's Story • The misadventures of **Harry Collins** – a young lad evacuated from his home in Stockport UK to Manitoba, Canada in WW2. 'An educational description of the life of an evacuee' **£9.95**

Just Visiting... • Charming and funny book by former Health Visitor **Molly Corbally**, who brilliantly depicts colourful characters and entertaining incidents from her long career. **£9.95**

Occupation Nurse • **Peter & Mary Birchenall** pay tribute to the achievement of the group of untrained nurses who provided healthcare at Guernsey's only hospital during the German occupation of 1940-45. **£9.95**

FICTION

A Trace of Calcium by **David Barnett** – A commuter comes to the aid of a young woman in trouble, becomes implicated in murder and must use all his resources to clear his name. **£9.95**

Double Time by **David Barnett** – A light-hearted time-travel fantasy in which a bookmaker tries to use a time machine to make his fortune and improve his love-life with hilarious consequences. **£9.95**

Last Sunset by **AA Painter** A nautical thriller set in the world of international yachting. A middle aged yachtsman becomes accidentally embroiled with smugglers, pirates and a very sexy young lady... **£9.95**

Retribution by **Mike Jupp** A very funny comedy/fantasy novel for adults and older children, featuring bizarre goings-on in a quiet English seaside town. Brilliantly illustrated. **£9.95**

The Cherkassy Incident by **Hunter Carlyle** A tense international thriller featuring a terrorist plot to steal nuclear missiles from a sunken Russian nuclear submarine. **£9.95**

MISCELLANEOUS SUBJECTS

Just a Butcher's Boy by **Christopher Bolton** Charming account of small town life in the 1950s in the rural Leiston, Suffolk and idyllic summers spent with grandparents who owned the local butcher's shop. **£5.95**

Impress of Eternity by **Paul McNamee** A personal investigation into the authenticity of the Turin Shroud. A former shcoolmaster examines the evidence and comes to a startling conclusion. **£5.95**

Making a Successful Best Man's Speech An indispensable aid to anyone who feels nervous about making a wedding speech. Tells you what to say and how to remember it. **£5.95**

Near & Yet So Far by **Audrey Truswell** The founder of an animal rescue charity tells charming and heart-warming tales of the rescue and rehabilitation of many four-legged friends in need. **£9.95**

Reputedly Haunted Inns of the Chilterns & Thames Valley by **Roger Long** – A light hearted look at pubs & the paranormal in the Heart of England **£5.95**

A Selection of London's Most Interesting Pubs by **David Gammell** – A personal selection of London's most unusual and historic hostelries with instructions how to find them. **£5.95**

Unknown to History and Fame by **Brenda Dixon** – Charming portrait of Victorian life in the West Sussex village of Walberton via the writings of Charles Ayling, a resident of the village, whose reports on local events were a popular feature in *The West Sussex Gazette* over many years during the Victorian era. **£9.95**

Woodfield books are available direct from the publishers by mail order as well as via all usual retail channels...

Telephone your orders to (**+44** if outside UK) **01243** 821234

Fax orders your to (**+44** if outside UK) **01243** 821757

All major credit cards accepted.

Visit our website for full details of all our titles – instant online ordering is also available at www.woodfieldpublishing.com

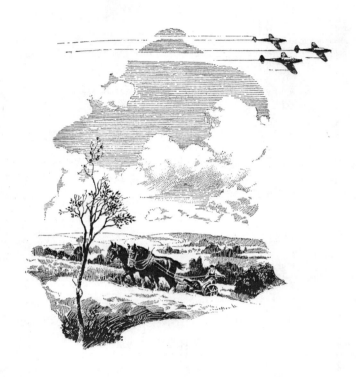

Woodfield Publishing
BABSHAM LANE ~ BOGNOR REGIS
WEST SUSSEX ~ ENGLAND
PO21 5EL

www.woodfieldpublishing.com